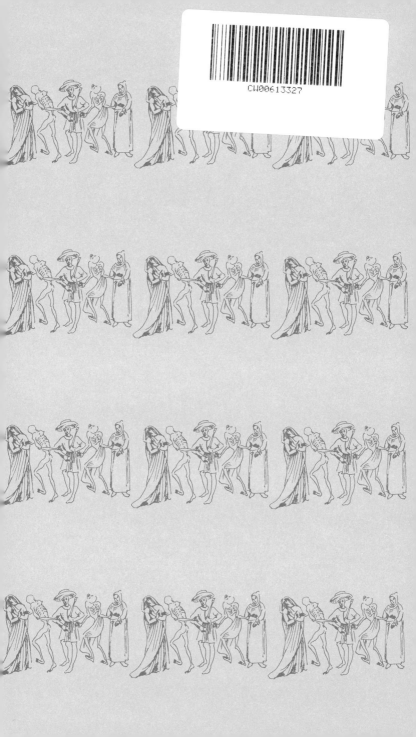

MEDICINE

THROUGH THE AGES

with Dr Baldassare

MEDICINE

THROUGH THE AGES

with Dr Baldassare

ROBERT RICHARDSON

Quiller Press

First published 1999 by Quiller Press Ltd,
46 Lillie Road, London, SW6 1TN
Copyright 1999 © Robert Richardson
The moral right of the author has been asserted

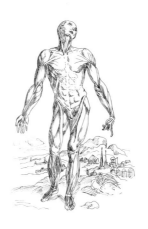

ISBN 1 899163 47 6

Illustrations by Michaela Gall
Jacket designed by Pat McCreeth
Book designed by Jo Lee
Set in Goudy 10pt on 12.5pt
Printed by Colorcraft Ltd. Hong Kong.

CONTENTS

Contents continued…

For Stella

Thou wert the morning star among the living,
Ere thy fair light had fled;
Now, having died, thou art as Hesperus, giving
New splendour to the dead.

Percy Bysshe Shelley, *To Stella* (from the Greek of Plato)

DR DAVID ANNANDALE'S
ENTANGLEMENT

James Grenfell sighed. It was a long academic sigh fading on the breath. It was an exquisitely controlled sigh, both in the depth of the inhalation and in the contemplation of the exhalation. It was a practised work of art. For his students, it had been a sign whose interpretation accorded with their degree of guilt, as it was never produced unless some moral dilemma had been brought to him for solution. For himself – he had once confided to me – it was no more and no less than an exercise to ensure that his lungs were working well, though he also admitted that the student's response was invariably enlightening. For me, now, sitting in his study drinking tea and hoping he did not regard me as a student again, it gave the lie to his own belief, since it seemed to breathe an understanding full of compassion. Maybe it was his eyes, searching deeply into mine, that gave the game away.

Professor James Grenfell had been my moral tutor at Oxford. He had long since been put out to grass in one of the college's cottages maintained for bachelor dons in their declining years, though there was nothing in decline about Grenfell. We still kept in touch and I would visit him whenever I had the sort of problem that other people might take to their vicar or astrologer – he was my guru. But this visit was like none of its predecessors as I had my doubts whether he would be able to help. Before his sigh, I had even wondered whether he would understand.

*   *   *

It is the not knowing that destroys the soul. Missing, believed… what? A witnessed death is a certain death. Either the spirit has moved on or there is total nothingness. Which you believe depends on your faith – or lack of it. Not for one moment do I believe Hester was killed in the plane crash; that would be too simple, too at variance with the circumstances of her previous existence. She continues, for good or ill, along the road mapped out by a perverse destiny. She may not be seen again in this life; but whenever that man chooses to call, she will be there. Though I loved her dearly, I was of no greater significance to her than a grain of sand lodged for a while in her shoe. Nevertheless, I am a grain of sand with feelings and I know I shall carry the burden of uncertainty to the grave.

In marrying Hester, I unwittingly became embroiled in the maelstrom that shaped two other lives. I was caught, tossed around and thrown back into a world that had lost its savour. But this is not my story, it is theirs – or rather his.

It all began, I suppose, some fifteen years ago. Hester and I had not been married long when something happened that shook us both rather badly. At the time we were living in an isolated hamlet above the Weald of Kent and our delight on a hot summer evening was to stroll hand-in-hand across the high fields. On this particular evening we seemed to be walking through patches of warm dry air – as if Nature had opened her oven door on to the windless sky. It was like nothing either of us had experienced before. I do not know whether it was just an ordinary meteorological phenomenon in those parts or whether it had some relevance to the events of the coming night, but I mention it because it created a wonderfully comfortable sensation and set us romanticizing about far away exotic places where lovers love for ever in the glow of eternal youth.

The sensation persisted as we lay in bed that night lost in our own silent dreams. When I awoke I felt as though I had slept deep and long, but the clock told me it was only just four and dawn was creeping up over the ridge on the far side of the valley. I put out a hand to touch Hester. The bed beside me was empty. A feeling of desperate urgency made me turn and I saw her standing in the open archway of the dressing room.

The force emanating from her was so elemental that it swamped my conscious sight with an utter blackness before the visual impulses had reached my thinking brain. In the same fragment of time I felt myself disintegrating in an all-consuming pain. My body was emotionally, physically and mentally paralysed. Yet something survived; I cannot explain what – perhaps it was the essential "me", my spirit, my soul. At all events, what happened next, what I saw, what I heard, what I breathed, was all experienced by that "me" and not by the me who is writing this. I no longer existed. The force surrounding Hester had both excluded me from its world and denied me my own.

I was not in my body, lying ignored on the bed, but floating freely somewhere above it all. How long the spectacle lasted I have no way of telling; like a dream it might have been over and done in an instant or, who knows, time might have been drawn out like a delicate thread to stretch the agony to breaking point. As Hester moved through the archway to stand for a moment motionless in the early light, I saw she was wearing a white cotton tunic held at the waist with a gold metal chain; on her wrists and ankles were ornate jewelled bracelets; her feet were bare.

The air was scented with a subtly insistent perfume. It had the freshness of spring, the fragrance of flowers at evening, the recollection of perfumes long forgotten. A delicate ethereal music filled the room. All that was beautiful was concentrated in and about her. "I" was being allowed a glimpse of the eternal woman.

Abruptly the spell was broken. The music ceased, the perfume dissolved, and Hester crumpled to the floor. Her tunic was torn from her by invisible hands, the bracelets turned to rings of blood and, as she lay there, a wound opened in her side and her life-blood ebbed away. At the sight I knew terrible desolation.

And that was when my sense of time played even stranger tricks. All I can do is set things down as I believe they happened. What was taking place, I realized afterwards, was a return to reality. The "me" that was out of my body began to weaken and as "I" faded I was aware of watching Hester lying on the floor in her pyjamas. Something akin to panic took over as "I" fought to get back into my body. I woke as my legs gave a final kick. The relief at finding myself back in my own world was tempered only by my concern for Hester, and here, fortunately, my conscious mind took over completely.

I got up – a bit groggily, I admit – and carried her back to bed. As I pulled the sheet up, she murmured something that sounded like

"Balshazzar" but so faintly I could not be sure. Having satisfied myself that she was deeply asleep and breathing comfortably, I climbed in beside her. I looked at the clock again – it was just after four.

I came to at my usual time of seven-thirty feeling perfectly normal – or as normal as it is possible for me to feel at that hour of the morning. Hester stirred.

"I'd love a cup of tea. I've got a bit of a head."

I padded off downstairs and, while waiting for the kettle to boil, started thinking. Despite a certain reluctance to accept it as such, the only reasonable conclusion I could reach was that I had had an incredibly vivid dream – heaven forbid that I had been hallucinating or that it had been an epileptic aura. That point more or less settled in my mind, I took our tea upstairs.

My confidence was sharply jolted when Hester reached out for her cup. Round her wrist the skin was rough and red – quite definitely so; nothing I could attribute to an overactive imagination.

"Hester, look at your wrist. How did that happen?" I put my cup on the table and sat beside her.

"Show me your other arm." Sure enough, her left wrist was in the same state.

"You've broken my dream." She spoke in a tense, almost frightened voice.

I opened my mouth to speak, but shut it again smartly.

"It was more of a nightmare than a dream," she went on after a moment or two. "But I really felt I was living through it – that it was really happening." And she then told me what I already knew, although quite a few of the details were missing. When she had finished I filled in those details for her. As I spoke I could sense the panic welling up inside her but she succeeded in keeping herself under control.

This proved to be the watershed. From then on we were both able to view the whole strange episode dispassionately and to discuss it like rational human beings.

By mutual I consent I began our attempt at analysis. "I saw your dream as clearly as I see you now. So what on earth can have been happening? Extrasensory perception can't be the answer – so much doesn't fit in. The marks on your wrists, for instance." And bending over to kiss those wrists, my heart missed a beat. Her pyjama top had fallen open and under her rib cage on her right side I could see a distinct red linear mark about three inches long. I touched it gently with my fingertips.

Hester twisted her head to see what I was doing. "I can't believe it!" She was now even more matter-of-fact than I. "It's sore, too. Look; there must be a logical explanation, otherwise we are going to find ourselves in incredibly deep waters. Could it be some sort of time warp or a time capsule – though whether they have any existence outside science fiction is beyond me. A spiritual explanation wouldn't really get us any further forward; accepting it would simply be an act of faith. My dream may be perfectly acceptable as a dream – but do we know what dreams are anyway? It's your seeing it as an outsider that puts the cat among the pigeons. And the way you saw it – the pain and the disembodiment. We could explain the disembodiment, perhaps, if we believed in spiritualism, but the pain is decidedly physical."

I was not going to argue with that. Indeed, the thought of a coronary had crossed my mind. "A heart attack in the here-and-now doesn't fill the bill – and anyhow I know I didn't have one. Whatever our explanation, it has to account for us both experiencing the same unreal occurrence and for its leaving those physical stigmas on you."

For the rest of the day we talked about little else. Lying in the sun for most of the time we let our minds roam, but a satisfactory explanation continued to elude us – as, in our heart-of-hearts, we knew was inevitable. I hesitate to think what the effect would have been, had we had even a glimmer of the true nature and implications of that experience.

It was when I reached this stage in my story that Grenfell sighed his sigh. He knew that Hester had left me, but only the bald fact, none of the circumstance. Yet I sensed that already he was far ahead of me and could account for the events of that night without knowing the sequel. I stopped to give him the opportunity of commenting, but he was content to hear me out.

"No, no, David my boy. Go on. You don't want an old fool interrupting with gratuitous irrelevancies before you have ended."

That was true enough – except that it would have been no old fool doing the interrupting.

I had not previously told the professor about the dream. Hester and I had regarded it simply as a strange experience shared between ourselves. Besides which the memory of it soon faded. Not quite to extinction, though; whenever I found myself in a library with a moment to spare I rooted about for anything that might give me a lead. But nothing appeared, despite my spreading the net widely from straight science, through the highways and byways of philosophy, metaphysics, magic, and history to religion and mythology.

Our lives, Hester's and mine, proceeded in an orderly fashion with, I would have said, more of the ups and fewer of the downs than afflict most human beings who chose to spend their lives together. We had no children, not because of any inability nor for any convoluted emotional reason – neither of us wanted them and we both felt we could get on well enough without. I, against much well-meaning advice, had gone into private medical practice and made a decent, though not spectacular, living; Hester did what she wanted to do which was to look after me and the home and generally help with the day-to-day running of the practice. We tended to take life as it came – and, to be honest, it came to us very comfortably.

In recent years I had been going to a number of international medical conferences, sometimes as just a delegate, at others as a speaker or as editor of the proceedings. It was a grand way to see the world and very few proved a disappointment. Hester nearly always came with me and, when practicable, we added a few days' sightseeing on our own.

In the spring of last year we went to a smallish meeting in Alexandria about yet another new antibiotic. More by chance than by design I had been associated with one of its clinical trials and had been asked to read a short paper. After the meeting we planned to spend a couple of days seeing Alexandria itself before taking the train to Cairo and making our way home from there.

The first morning on our own we were up early and, with Hester in charge of the guide-book, set out to explore the city. From our hotel we headed for the Eastern Harbour and came on the magnificent sweeping corniche at the southernmost part of its curve. At that hour it was breathtaking in its freshness; in fact, it reminded me more of a northern Mediterranean coast than of Africa – an impression borne out by the people, too. We strolled along Sharia 26 July with the sun warming our backs and turning the rooftops of the dun brown facades almost white in the morning air. Passing more quickly through the seedy El Anfushi quarter we came to Fort Qabay, built on the foundations of Alexander the Great's Pharos – it is indeed partly built of marble from that lighthouse. Until that moment my mind had been absorbed with the pleasures of a modern day in a modern city, but as I touched the stone I felt the past quivering under my fingers. The marble had been quarried two and a half thousand years ago on the orders of a man as he set out to conquer the world. From the summit of the double storied tower a great fire had blazed out at night to guide ships safely into harbour.

I was brought back to the present by Hester's voice. "We just go back the way we came and keep going."

"What?" I said. "I'm sorry, I was miles away dreaming about Alexander and his lighthouse."

"And I was dreaming about the man himself. Just think what he achieved. He was only thirty-two when he died. Do you know where he was buried?" Hester was deep into the guide-book. "I'd always thought it was in Babylon, but it says here that his body was brought to Alexandria and buried at the crossroads of the ancient world. I want to go there, David; it sounds so romantic and exciting. Imagine being able to throw your cloak on the ground and have an architect build a city to its shape with the centre street a hundred feet wide."

As we started to retrace our steps, I had an unpleasant sense of foreboding; it was one of those irrational feelings that descend out of the blue and is completely at odds with the day. If anything, it was, I suppose, like the feeling of dread that used to afflict me on the way back to prep school at the start of a new term. Fortunately, it seemed not to be catching and Hester was bubbling along excitedly beside me. Having exhausted what the guide-book had to say about Alexander the Great, she gave a little skip and grasped hold of my hand.

"Oh! darling, I'm so happy. I haven't enjoyed one of these trips so much for ages."

She looked up at me and, despite my mental overcast, I responded. How could I have done otherwise? Her eyes were sparkling with happiness and her whole face was aglow with delight. There, in the middle of a street in Alexandria, I stopped, put my arms around her and kissed her.

"I love you. Always remember I love you."

My spirits lifted and, hands held tightly together, we walked on, scorning the curious looks of the passers-by.

Shortly afterwards we found ourselves in the Sharia Nebi Danyal which, the guide-book informed us, had been named not after the prophet Daniel but after one Muhamed Danyal al-Maridi who had died in comparatively recent times in 1407. The point where this street had crossed the Canopic Way in Alexander's city had been the crossroads of the world. Now, the Canopic Way is the more prosaic sounding Sharia el Mitwalli to the west and Sharia Horreya to the east. Where the crossroads of the modern world might be is anybody's guess.

A few yards past the crossing is the mosque where Nebi Danyal once preached – though the present building is nineteenth-century – and it marks the site of Alexander's tomb. We were standing in the shade of the building opposite studying the guide-book when, for the second time in my life I became an impotent observer of the inexplicable – only this time I was not the spectator of another's dream, I was seeing my own life fall apart.

I had looked at my watch to see whether we should have a coffee before or after visiting the mosque. It was a minute or two after ten-thirty. Hester was staring across the road at the mosque. I touched her arm to attract her attention. The power that hit me was indescribable. As far as I can recall them, the sensations I experienced on the first occasion were repeated. Above all, there was the terrifying pain – I felt I must have been screaming with the agony of it – which accompanied the dissolution of my body. But, as before something survived and, from above Sharia Nebi Danyal at ten-thirty on a perfect spring morning, "I" looked down on myself leaning against the wall, to all intents and purposes casually studying a guide-book. Yet it was not my own behaviour I was concerned with, it was Hester's.

A diminutive Arab boy had materialized at her side. In answer to his tug at her skirt, she took both his hands in hers and kissed him on the brow. Never in my life had I seen a kiss so devoid of sensuality, yet so full of affection. No mother ever kissed her child with so pure an emotion; in every mother's love for her offspring is an element of sexuality whether she accepts it or not. Here was something unique, born out of this world and bearing deep in its heart an aura of timelessness. The little figure in its immaculate white burnous beamed with joy before pulling at Hester's hands.

"Come. He is waiting," he said. And together they crossed to the other side of the street, traffic and pedestrians parting like the Red Sea.

Though my recollection of the incidental, normal everyday

happenings is blurred in the extreme, that of the meeting between Hester and Dr Paul Baldassare will be engraved on my memory for as long as I live. Again the energy surrounding Hester excluded me from whatever world she had entered. Again I was temporarily an outcast from my own. Time was without its foundation.

As Hester and the boy reached the opposite side, a man stepped towards them. He was dressed in an exquisitely cut light grey suit with hand-made shoes; his tie was of plain blue silk and his shirt had unquestionably come from Bond Street. He was just under six foot tall and well-proportioned. Only the slightest hint of thickening around his waist gave me a clue to his age. He must have been over fifty, though he moved like a fit and very much younger man. His colouring was in complete contrast to that of the fair, blue-eyed Hester; he was dark with thick brown-black hair flecked with grey at the temples. His strong regular features, his bearing, his manner, all spoke of strength of character.

He stood there with his arms open. "Hester!"

The way he said her name made it sound like "Ishtar". It was floated lovingly like the merest zephyr; it was quite the most beautiful of names. As I watched, Hester's face, already exquisite enough to turn any man's head, was transfigured.

For a moment they stood still, glorying in each other's presence. Then Hester was in his arms and they kissed. It was a kiss that defied the boundaries of eternity. It had a timelessness as though with this kiss the world had been born and with it, too, the world would die. I was not watching two people lost in an embrace, but one spirit lost in the contemplation of its immortality.

I saw no more. Suddenly "I" found myself spinning giddily into blackness.

"A door in the north-west wall leads to an arcaded courtyard. Inside the mosque, seven arcades running parallel to the kiblah (the direction in which Mohammedans turn to pray) support the wooden roof. The cellars and crypt have never been properly excavated." I raised my eyes from the guide-book and looked at my watch. It was a minute or two after ten-thirty.

"Hester!" I could see where she and the man had been standing but now they were gone. As an icy cold fear crept into my bones, I felt someone gently tweaking my sleeve. It was the immaculate little Arab boy. "Baksheesh" I thought. I pulled out a coin, any coin, from my pocket and gave it to him.

"No Sir, I do not ask for money." His English was as immaculate as his dress. "I have come with a message. My master wishes me to ensure no harm comes to you."

The wave of fear receded, only to be replaced by complete and utter bewilderment. What had happened to Hester? Who was this strange boy? Though perhaps more pertinently, who was his master? The questions kept tumbling over each other, but the presence of the boy at my side seemed, in some inexplicable manner, to calm my torment.

"Dr Annandale, Sir." How did he know my name? "I think we should return to your hotel before I answer your questions." Could he read my mind as well? "I shall explain everything then." And, almost as an afterthought, he added, "Your wife is perfectly safe."

Together we walked the short distance to the hotel discussing, of all things, the cultural implications of Napoleon's occupation of Egypt, a subject on which he seemed surprisingly well informed. The possibility that I should be looking for Hester never once occurred to me. At the hotel, he asked for my key by its correct number and ordered a light lunch to be served in my room.

My wife had disappeared in a Middle-Eastern city and here was I sitting calmly in a hotel bedroom, quite unconcerned about the affair, talking to the Arab servant of the man responsible for her abduction. Even now I cannot believe I did nothing for a whole fortnight, but that was the case. The fact that I was in a delirium for most of the time is a poor excuse for my lack of action on that first day. But I was not behaving rationally even then – that must be obvious to the least generous minded. The only explanation I can adduce is that the power of this boy, or his master, over my mind must have been absolute. I was *made* to do nothing. I was *made* not to care about the person I held most dear in all the world.

When lunch arrived, the Arab dismissed the waiter and himself laid up the meal on the desk-cum-dressing table. Having finished his task, he turned round and pulled back the hood of his burnous. To my astonishment, he was not an Arab at all. He was fair, very fair, with the most extraordinarily crisp, curly golden hair and striking blue eyes; his nose would probably best be described as snub, and his chin and the tips of his ears as pointed. His expression was that of a mischievous pixie, though as he searched my face there was only sympathy in his gaze. He must also have been considerably older than I had imagined.

"Who on earth are you?" I blurted out. "You're not an Arab, are you?"

"No, Dr Annandale, I am not an Arab." He took no offence at my rudeness. "Originally, I am a Greek and my name is Telesphorus."

"So your master is also a Greek?" I hazarded.

"No: originally he was a..." he hesitated, "an Iraqi." I could see I was going to have to work for my information.

"Why do you say originally? What nationality are you now?"

"Ah!" He smiled a cherubic smile. "You English do love to put everyone in their correct pigeonhole. My master was born in what is now Iraq and I was born on the slopes of Mount Olympus – nothing can change those facts. But, in truth, we are both cosmopolitans."

I chose to let pass his assumption that I was English: I am a Scot. "And who is this master of yours?"

"Dr Paul Baldassare." It was said with pride, as if to be the servant of the man were honour enough. Indeed such seemed to be the case, for at that moment there was a knock at the door and a deferential manager entered.

"Excuse me, Sir," he bowed towards me, "I have a note for Mr Telesphorus."

I nodded my permission.

"From Dr Baldassare," he said as he handed the letter to Telesphorus. "If there is a reply...?"

"By your leave?" Telesphorus inclined his golden head. I nodded again. Whatever his nationality, he could only have been educated at an English public school! He read the note at a glance.

"Thank you; there is no reply." And I would swear that the manager must still have been walking backwards and bowing when he reached his foyer.

"Now, if you will eat, I shall answer your questions." With a sweeping gesture he gathered up a chair and deposited it at the desk. "My master – that note was from him – and mistress have left Alexandria. I am to follow as soon as I know you will come to no harm."

This reference to "my mistress" was obviously to Hester, yet I felt not the slightest concern. For all the emotional impact the news had upon me, he might as well have been announcing that two close friends had gone on holiday. If I had needed further proof that my world was being turned upside down and that I had lost control of my destiny, I had it then.

"Why should I come to harm?" The lunch was delicious. "Aren't you eating?" I waved my fork in his direction.

"No, I do not eat when there is work to be done." Although his voice was soft and kind, he was chiding me ever so gently for not concentrating on the really important matter – but that was his fault, not mine. "You asked why you might come to harm. The answer is one I do not expect you to understand – or not without help. You have, most regrettably, been caught up in a slight miscalculation of timing in the eternal ordering of events – forgive me if I sound unduly dramatic – and we have to ensure that neither your spirit nor your body suffers any permanent hurt as a result. Your mind might become unhinged – forgive me again. You might contemplate taking your own life when you discovered your wife had left you without hope of her return. You must accept that you will never see her again; but whether you do or not will make no difference. She and my master are gone for ever. All I can do is make this episode in your life as painless as it lies in my power to do."

With that he took both my hands in his, looked me straight in the eye, and began to recite what I must assume to have been a prayer. I did not hear its end. I had taken about as much as it is reasonable to expect any man to take without cracking – and I cracked.

The next fourteen days are lost to me. I have only the hotel manager's account to go on, and it was all very simple: "Dr Annandale has been ill. But what a fortunate man he was to have Dr Baldassare's servant look after his needs. Mr Telesphorus insisted on doing everything himself; he would accept no help from the hotel. If it had been anyone other than Mr Telesphorus, I would have sent Dr Annandale to hospital."

"Where is Mr Telesphorus now?" I asked.

"He took his departure this morning. He settled your account in full and for a further week. By then, he assured us, you would be fully recovered and able to leave." He would not be sorry to see me go. It was further testimony to the influence of Dr Baldassare that the presence of a sick man in the hotel had been endured for fourteen days. I was about to enquire whether he knew anything of my wife's whereabouts when he forestalled me.

"Mr Telesphorus asked me to inform you that your wife was travelling home with Dr Baldassare and that you were aware of the arrangements."

I turned away from him as the tears welled in my eyes.

Deep within me I knew that what Telesphorus had said about Hester and this Dr Baldassare was the truth. I might not understand why it was the truth, but that was irrelevant. What was not irrelevant were my emotions. I could not – I would not – leave Egypt without making some attempt to find out what had really happened.

My strength returned rapidly. Before venturing outside, I telephoned my secretary who, to my surprise, asked how I was and whether I would still be coming home at the end of the week. It appeared that I had already telephoned her some days previously to say I was unwell and to cancel my appointments until further notice. Mr Telesphorus thought of everything.

That week was the most frantic of my life. I shall not go into the details of the search; let it suffice that as time went on and I questioned more and more people, the further away I knew I was getting. The police were sympathetic, but quite obviously if a woman had left her husband for another man…. The shrug of the shoulders said it all. No one at the Faculty of Medicine at the University had ever heard of Dr Baldassare and my quizzing of the hotel manager elicited only the information that the doctor had been staying at the hotel with his servant and had left on the day of my arrival. The good doctor certainly knew how to influence people even if he won few friends in the process.

On my last day, I picked up an English language newspaper. A headline on the front page caught my eye: MYSTERY PLANE CRASH IN DESERT. The story was short.

"Three people are believed to have been killed when a light aircraft crashed in the desert near the Siwa oasis. The body of the pilot, who has not yet been named, was found in the burnt out wreckage. There was no trace of the passengers. The plane had been chartered by an Iraqi doctor. He was accompanied by a woman who is understood to be British. The possibility that the aircraft violated Libyan airspace and was shot down by a Libyan airforce jet is strongly denied by the Libyan authorities."

It had to be them.

I immediately tried to charter a plane myself, but when I mentioned

Siwa my request was met with obstinate refusal. Siwa was in a militarily restricted area and off limits to foreigners. I knew when I was beaten.

The next morning, on my way past the Reception desk, the manager beckoned me. "I have this package for you. It was left by Mr Telesphorus to be given you on your departure." As the parcel was quite heavy, I put it in one of my cases – there was plenty of room; all Hester's clothes and belongings had vanished while I was ill.

When I arrived home, my first thought was to contact James Grenfell to see what he would make of my bizarre tale and to seek his advice on how to deal with my shattered private life. He told me to come as soon as I liked and to stay for a long as I liked. My second thought was to open Telesphorus's package. It proved to contain a number of folders crammed with sheets of paper. There was a covering letter from Dr Baldassare.

"Dear Doctor Annandale," it read. "I make no apologies for my actions. Ishtar is mine and always will be. This manuscript is my autobiography and, as with many works of its kind, it is well informed by hindsight. It is not the first time I have written the story and I doubt it will be the last. When you have read it, I hope you will find it in your heart to feel pity for me." It was signed, "Paul Baldassare". There was no address and no date.

I then turned my attention to the folders. What I read in the pages sent me racing off to James. I was too emotionally involved in the last episode to be able to take a dispassionate view of the whole. I did not know whether to believe the story or not – and I felt a desperate need to know. That was why I had to have James's impartial judgment.

When I had told him my tale, I handed him the letter and the folders.

DR PAUL BALDASSARE'S STORY

1

"You must learn that disease is not a divine affliction" *

My memories of childhood are irretrievably blurred. As the centuries slipped away, those years congealed into one amorphous day that began with the hour of my birth in the city of Kish in the land of Akkad. And it was, indeed, a very long time ago.

You would not now recognize my Kish. The mighty Euphrates, which brought our trade and gave us our prosperity, has changed its course, not once but many times. In my youth, the river flowed hesitantly past the mud-brick walls of the city. My home lay within those walls, barely distinguishable from the many thousands of others and dominated, even then, by temples and the ziggurat. Outside were gardens, rich with magnolia and rhododendron, cotoneaster and berberis, anemone and fritillaria ranged among sweet smelling herbs; further away we grew our fruits and vegetables and, further away still, flocks of sheep and cattle grazed close by fields of barley, wheat and millet – all nourished by the interlacing canals and ditches dug with such skill by our forefathers. Beneath the walls themselves and convenient to the gates of the city

* For one reason or another Dr Baldassare has given no dates in his story. Whether this is because he cannot remember them or because he expects you to know from the historical context, is anybody's guess. I rather suspect that, for his peace of mind, he wished to compress time so that, while writing, he could simply view his life on the same scale as we would ours. Nevertheless, I thought it advisable to give the dates of the period covered at the start of each chapter; thus the events in this first part of Dr Baldassare's story took place roughly between 2700 BC and 1500 BC. At David Annandale's request I have also appended a dated listing of the characters he mentions. – J.G.

lay the harbour full of craft busy with trade to the cities of the north and to Sumer and the world beyond in the south. Kish was then the seat of kingship and our ruler held supremacy over both Akkad and Sumer, countries that a millennium-and-a-half later together became Babylonia. Bab-ilim itself, some fifty miles to the west, was still a desert village of which few had heard and remarkable only for its insignificance. Yet the errant waters were to bring her greatness and an immortality peculiar in the romance of history. [This, Dr Annandale, is perhaps why I like to think of myself as a Babylonian – and who is there now that would challenge my assumption?]*

*   *   *

My father was a merchant in the city. He was rich but others were richer and that displeased him. It was this avaricious nature of his that was indirectly responsible for my future predicament and directly so for his own death. Not content with the well-earned comforts of home and the respect of the citizens, he had to listen to travellers' tales of awesome wealth waiting to be gathered in from distant places. If he had only listened and contented himself with dreaming... but no, he was suddenly taken with the urge to see and gather in for himself. That was bad enough; what made it a disaster was his determination to take me, his eldest son, with him. I was then, if I recall correctly, in my sixteenth year and had completed my schooling at the tablet house. My father could not be made to see that if riches were there for the taking in Nubia's golden mountains, why in the name of Anu did these tellers of tales come scratching at his door begging for food and shelter. No amount of pleading by either my mother (admittedly half-hearted) or myself would shake him from his decision – he was determined, as he expressed it, to complete my education. I was developing other ideas of how to achieve that same end.

As the day of departure drew nearer, my father spent more and more time in one of the temples. Much incense was burned and many sheep slaughtered that their entrails might be staked out to reveal the fate of the expedition. The omens were consistently good – did not my father contribute handsomely to the welfare of the priests? But I knew

* The typescript contained many comments scribbled by Dr Baldassare evidently for David Annandale's benefit. Some I found almost indecipherable. – J.G.

better. How I knew better was simple: my intelligence (in more than one sense of the word) was better. My mother, still a strikingly beautiful woman, had made all her decisions in recent years on the advice of an esteemed diviner at whose house she was a frequent and welcomed visitor. Her scheme worked well enough until the breaking of my voice had opened my eyes to the ways of the world. I knew there was profit lurking somewhere in my new-found discovery, if I was content to bide my time. I was, and the time had come.

I visited Ebih-Il, for that was his name, and put my proposition to him: he would interpret truly the omens governing the expedition – and more particularly, my part in it – or I would immediately inform my father of my mother's infidelity. His response left me totally nonplussed.

"He already knows." His smile was quite open. "But even so I will see what the future holds for you, if..." the smile broadened as he watched my discomfiture develop, "...if you will acquire for me the little statue of the god Abu that is your father's."

Of course I stole the wretched thing and brought it to him a few days later.

He made me stand before him like a child, the spirit seething within me at the man's insolence. "You were a fool, Bal-sarra-uzur, to believe me. But I shall keep to my side of our bargain, if only to teach you a lesson." He gave me a very strange penetrating look before walking across to the window overlooking the river and began to intone. "I have offered incense and observed the oil and the water; I have summoned Ishtar, the Bringer of Dawn...." Suddenly he stopped and, with an overly dramatic gesture, brought the flat of his hand to his brow. Sinking slowly to the ground, he murmured: "The mist closes about me and has shut the future from my eyes!" As his body touched the ground it seemed, to my overwrought imagination, that it settled itself comfortably before lying motionless. Even diviners can come to an unexpectedly abrupt end if the gods choose to send death to visit them. There was only one sensible thing for me to do – and I did it. I picked up my father's little statue and hurried home.

I make no secret of my terror. Beyond doubt I was doomed. For Ebih-Il to be called away when about to disclose the revelations of Ishtar opened the gateway to a perplexing array of omens. Inanna-Ishtar, child of the Moon god, the Morning and the Evening star, was also goddess of war and goddess of love. She was supposed to be the comforter of man but, riding astride her sacred lion, in either of her aspects she could bring him to glory or destruction. I had little doubt which she had in mind for me.

My mother tore at her favourite green robe – the one she wore for her illicit visits – took to her couch and refused to rise. My father lost patience with her, pointing out that other merchants had journeyed far afield to return safely and endow their wives with great joy and comfort. (He was not to know that the cause of my mother's distress lay quite elsewhere.) I gained reassurance from the knowledge that Ebih-Il had been a liar and a deceiver as I now believed his divination, whatever it was, would have been worthless and that he had paid the price of his iniquity.

Soon my father's boats were fully loaded, some with barley, wheat, dates, fish oil, wool and skins for barter along the way; others, carefully disguised with objects of no worth, were filled with statuettes and heads of copper and bronze; figurines in polished black stone; necklaces and bracelets of gold inset with agate beads; silver bars; glass drinking vessels and much else besides of great beauty and value made from materials acquired on previous, less hazardous, journeys. He was staking his present wealth against a dream of untold riches. Oh! gullible and foolish man.

But where there is trade, there also is corruption. Whether by accident or whether by subornation – I suspect the latter – our head boatman led us astray from the main channel and into the marshes of Sumer when we had passed by Ur. He said he was lost and would set out to find a guide. That night we were attacked. My father and many of his servants were slaughtered – my mother would now have real cause to grieve – while those of us who survived were stripped and put in neck stocks; there was to be no escape.

At daylight, our captors examined us carefully. When they came to me, I stared at them in defiance. But instead of humiliating me as they had the others, I saw fear enter into them and they began arguing amongst themselves. At last they reached a decision and one of them – their leader, I imagine – took my head between his hands and gazed at me in wonder before falling to his knees to kiss my feet while another removed my stock. My garments and sandals were returned and I was given food to eat and beer to drink.

I have an aptitude for tongues and had acquired a few words of Sumerian from visitors to my father's house; consequently I was able to follow the substance of these people's talk. It seems they believed the colour of my eyes gave me the magical power to penetrate the secrets of the universe. For my eyes are blue, a blue as deep and intense as the sky at midday and enough to strike wonder into the minds of the superstitious and ignorant. Among my own people, this gift of Nature was rare, but not unique, and appeared, so I had been told, from time to time among those with ancestors whose seed, by one means or another, had found its way to Akkad from distant northern lands.

My recollection of the events of the next months – or it may have been years, I have no means of telling – is confused in all respects. Suffice it to say that I was passed from people to people and from country to country until eventually I found myself in Memphis in the hands of an ambitious nobleman who had acquired me with one intention only – the hope of advancement by presenting me to the king's vizier as a gift. Slaves from Kish were always in demand on account of our intellectual abilities, and the opportunity of finding one as young and as unusual as myself, arose but rarely. I was indeed a gift to be treasured.

The king's vizier, Imhotep by name, was possessed of more talents than any man has a right to expect. I shall not speak of his genius as architect and builder; time has done that for me as it is there for all to see in the shape of his monument, the pyramid and last resting place of his master, the Pharaoh Zoser. It may be a ruin now, but when I first saw it, it was gloriously encased in dressed stone and, with its vast white-panelled enclosing wall, stunned the eye from every corner of Memphis. Neither shall I speak of his wisdom, reflected in his capacity as High Priest of Heliopolis and Recorder of Judgments, nor of his knowledge of the movements of the stars. But I shall speak of his understanding of the ills suffered by mankind – though at the time I was greatly puzzled by his denial of divine intervention.

Imhotep's compassionate nature was reflected in his broad and kindly face, his strengths in a firm mouth and chin. He treated me more like a son than a slave and was greatly concerned to continue my education. I found no difficulty with his teaching of mathematics as in Akkad we were already adepts; nor with his teaching of astronomy once he had persuaded me to abandon the astrological overtones we had introduced at home. No, it was something quite otherwise that my mind would not accept. In Akkad we believed that sickness and death were brought by the gods or by malignant jinn. That was why Ebih-Il had wanted my father's little statue of Abu; the image of the god was hard to come by, but the protection it could give was fearsome though not, as Ebih-Il discovered, when dishonestly obtained. I argued from the analogy of a gift: when one person gives something to another, the gift is a thing apart from both. Yet, try as I might, I could not persuade Imhotep of the truth of our beliefs.

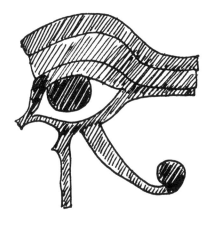

The eye of Horus. This is said to be the origin of the recipe symbol (R) that is written at the start of medical prescriptions. The eye formed the design for a powerful amulet in Ancient Egypt. In the sometimes confused mythology of the times, Horus - besides being a major deity whose eyes were torn out by Seth, but had his sight restored by the healing god, Thot - is often referred to as a physician.

Imhotep studied me closely for a moment or two, no doubt deciding whether, after all, I was worthy of his continued effort.

"In your country," he said at last, "the priests study the entrails of animals to forecast the future?" It was a question. I nodded, sullenly. "When the livers are smooth and shiny, the omens are good?" I nodded again. "And when they are shrunken, discoloured, hard or knobbly, the omens are bad?" I bowed my head in assent. "These animals are afflicted," he continued, "not by a thing apart but by disease that has entered their bodies as an instrument of destruction. The priests can see this, even though they do not understand.

"The gods do, indeed, have powers to govern what we are; but much may happen in our lives over which they have no influence. You must learn that disease is not a divine affliction, but has causes that one day we shall understand. In my lifetime, I shall be able to do little more than look at a man who is sick and try to give what comfort I can." He sighed in despair at his helplessness. "When we know the causes and can observe their effects, then shall we be able to judge whether to treat or not."

It would be many centuries before mankind again saw the healing art with Imhotep's clarity of vision. But at that time, when I stood beside him gazing at his homage to eternity, I could see only an old man whose brain was becoming addled like an egg that has been kept too long. When the gods are denied, they will surely seek to destroy.

I thought I might disconcert him by asking where he had gained his knowledge. "Through Thoth was I instructed in the mysteries of SA-HA-Hor, the protection round the falcon, where our Child of the Sun shall rest on his journey to paradise in the sky." As good an answer as any, I suppose, and one that showed he did believe in divine wisdom. And in all the years since, I have never heard a better explanation of the origin of knowledge. It will forever remain a closed book.

Imhotep wrote of the sick and injured who were brought to him; I earnestly prayed these papyri would never fall into the hands of the pharaoh – such sacrilege would bring swift retribution, whoever the perpetrator. When he felt powerless to help, Imhotep wrote that the man was to be left untreated or "moored at his mooring stakes until the period of his injury passes by", a quaint phrase, but typical of the man in his whimsical moods.

There were occasions, nevertheless, when he would bring about a cure and I would watch in fascination while he straightened a broken bone before holding the limb firm with slats of wood bound with linen and stiffened with gums.

I watched him, too, save wounds from rotting by washing them with willow water; small ones he then closed by pulling together with gummed linen, though the ones that gaped he stitched as you would a rent garment. On the first day he bound fresh meat over the wound; thereafter, an ointment of grease and honey sufficed.

Imhotep was wise in many other respects which I did not understand until long years afterwards. He knew that the pulse, which he could feel in different parts of the body, was related to the motions of the heart. He also understood that severe blows to the head or spine could cause paralysis, deafness, incontinence and other disorders. All this he wrote down.

Yet, despite the evidence of my own eyes, I still did not believe him and made my disbelief plain. I refused to help him, saying that by doing so I would offend my gods. I could no more interfere with their work than I could command the rain to fall, the wind to blow or the rocks to stem the river's flow.

When I had been with Imhotep for about two years and he still could not persuade me to his way of thinking – I refused stubbornly to be shaken from beliefs which had been instilled into me from childhood – he gave me, one day at our morning meal, a pleasant-tasting drink which, he said, would grant me insight into a matter of great importance.

"Bal-sarra-uzur, today we shall go to the temple where you must decide your fate. I shall ask you a question: 'Do you wish to stay on earth until mankind comes to understand the nature of disease?'" This seemed a strange question. After all, except for Imhotep, mankind already knew that disease came from the gods. My perplexity must have been evident. "You wonder why I should ask such a question? That is for you to discover. Your answer must depend on your beliefs."

Suddenly at that moment, I felt my life to be a dream. As the day progressed, its events floated in and out of that dream. How much was real and how much enchantment, I cannot say as the drink had undoubtedly made me hallucinate.

"Remember, Bal-sarra-uzur, if you wish to discover the answer, it will be a long time coming." Those were the last words I am certain I heard him speak.

*   *   *

At the entrance to the temple we were met by two priests. In my dream-like world I passed down long passages lit only by the light entering from small windows set high in the walls, through rooms where alabaster oil lamps suspended on the columns fluttered in the draught. The corridors were bare of furnishings but in the many halls stood golden altars and beautifully worked statues. The walls were covered with panels depicting day-to-day life. And wherever I looked, shaven-headed priests in their long linen robes were going about their duties.

"Wait," Imhotep instructed me in a voice that came from far away. "When the great door opens, pass through. I shall be ready to greet you." With that, he and the two priests left me.

The door at the end of the corridor where I was standing was massive and delicately worked in gold. On its far side lay the great hall of the temple. Already I could hear the chanting of the priests as they gathered there – or was the sound in my imagination? I believed I was about to be sacrificed and I welcomed the thought. Obeying the call of my gods seemed to be the only way to convince Imhotep that they were the masters of disease. I calmly decided I would answer: "Yes, I wish to stay."

Slowly the great doors parted. I remained motionless until they had swung back to their full extent and I could see every detail of the hall – but it was like nothing remembered. In the centre was a small pool with, at the far end, a fountain bubbling out of the mouth of a crocodile skilfully carved from the stone. The hall was circular and two paces in from the walls was a ring of fluted columns. The walls themselves were covered with reliefs of various sports played along the river's banks. There were no windows; as with the halls I had passed through all the light came from oil lamps. Chairs, tables and couches were grouped around the floor. Opposite me, on the other side of the pool, Imhotep sat on a carved throne, inlaid with gold, silver and ivory, and raised on four steps.

I scarcely trusted my legs to carry me as I walked forward round the water's edge, and on towards the steps. I knelt and placed my brow on the lowermost. The chanting had stopped.

"Bal-sarra-uzur, you have been brought here for Imhotep to question you." A disembodied voice filled the hall. "Have you decided what your answer shall be?"

I rose and bowed deeply.

Imhotep, unfamiliar in the ibis-head mask he wore in his capacity of Recorder of Judgments, inclined his head.

"Bal-sarra-uzur, we have spoken together. Do you wish to continue on earth until mankind understands the nature of disease?"

While he spoke I almost believed he was truly inspired by Re and all the gods of Egypt. Beneath the beak-headed mask I could see his face, transfigured. It was as though he already knew the answer I would give.

I bowed deeply once again. As I raised my head I looked into his eyes. His pupils dilated and contracted in a steady rhythm; then they began to spin, faster and faster, larger and larger, bearing down upon me, relentlessly seeking to enter my own. The world around me filled with their motion until I also began to spin. Faster and faster I went, still with those two points of blackness before me, pulsing and ebbing, pulsing and ebbing, spinning ever faster and faster.

Suddenly they became as two blinding orbs of light. All movement ceased and with it my spirit left my body to soar floating in blessed tranquillity. As from afar I heard a voice: "Then I fear it will be for ever."

So this was death!

But as my spirit watched and listened, life on earth continued.

"Eternal life has been granted; eternal life shall be taken!" And Imhotep struck two blows on the gong at his side.

The door behind him opened, and the renewed singing of the priests and the playing of harpists filled the air. Through the door came a young priestess wrapped in a cloak the colour of the sky when the sun has set and fastened about her throat with a golden clasp. Slowly she walked to the foot of the steps where my lifeless body lay. Gazing down at me she unloosed the clasp and with a graceful sweep of her arm spread the cloak in a circle on the floor. On its inner side, now exposed to view, were mystical designs woven in delicate silver tracery. She stepped back. Beneath the gauzy veils, held at the waist by a gold-worked belt, her body glistened. About her wrists and ankles were jewelled bracelets, and in her navel there nestled a jewel set in gold.

She began to dance. Her body quivered beneath the veiling as she swayed back and forth, from side to side, her arms never still, weaving a sinuous pattern. On and on she danced, rising towards a climax, falling away again, but ever moving onwards into ecstasy. The end came with a terrifying suddenness as she fell across the cloak, distorting its symbolism, and lay motionless. Then she raised herself and kissed me on the brow. With that kiss my spirit was drawn back into my body.

Still unable to move I watched the two priests enter and brutally tear the bracelets from her wrists and ankles, leaving in their stead circlets of blood. Then one stepped forward, ceremonial sword in hand. For several moments he stood above her, intoning rapidly to himself. I did not see the sword pierce her side.

But I heard her cry and looked up at her. She smiled. This girl who was dying smiled at me.

"Bal-sarra-uzur, I am very near death. Kiss me, that we may meet again."

With strength flowing back to me, even as it left her body, I turned my head and kissed her lips.

The kiss was broken by death.

"Bal-sarra-uzur." It was Imhotep who spoke. "She was a priestess of Astarte, who in your country you know as Ishtar!"

*　　*　　*

If you wish to dismiss this as nothing more than fantasy, the product of a disordered hallucinating mind, so be it. I can only assure you that it – or something closely resembling what I have described – did indeed happen. But, as I have said, it was all a very long time ago.

In the early years, I was myself sceptical that anything had happened. I remained Imhotep's chosen slave and was by his side when he died, leaving me in the charge of a priest-physician to care for the sick – in which respect my beliefs were unchanged and now not even challenged. Imhotep's heretical ideas about disease were, like his writings, lost to sight.

With the passing years, my body showed none of the signs of age; it retained its resilience and strength. Men looked at me strangely and began to avoid my company. When my new master also died, I slipped away from the temple and joined the river traders. I moved from boat to boat until eventually I became my own master. Nevertheless, I learned not to remain in one place for too long – I was stoned through the gates of more than one city. Time grew meaningless; perhaps the gods took pity on me as, alone in desert places, I would occasionally fall asleep in some natural shelter only to wake decades, maybe centuries, later refreshed and ready to journey on. Invariably, so it seemed in those days, the world and its people did not change.

In the reign of Amenophis I, I was working in the temple of Ammon-Re in Karnak as an assistant scribe to Seneb, a priest-physician and keeper of the papyri, one of whose tasks was to record the remedies used in the House of Life. Regrettably, the healers in these Houses relied closely on what was contained in their cases of writings.

"See, Bal-sarra-uzur," Seneb called to me in his excitable manner, "here is an ancient papyrus from the ruins in Memphis."

I went over to him and started reading. The writing was, without doubt, in the hand of Imhotep. My heart beat faster and a lump came to my throat as I touched the ancient papyrus, my head full of memories. Seneb obviously did not appreciate the significance of what he was copying* – if, indeed, he understood the hieroglyphs. With considerable self-restraint, I refrained from naming the author. My knowledge would only lead to the asking of unanswerable questions, the more particularly as Imhotep's fame now rested on his architectural achievements.

"By the bye," Seneb stopped writing and looked up at me. "I learnt a number of new incantations today. They expel the sickness of the year gone by, and grant protection for the one that is to come." So saying, he turned over the papyrus on which he was writing and began again on the back**, speaking the words as he wrote: "O Flame-in-his-Face! Presider over the Horizon, speak thou to the Chief of the Hemesut House who makes Osiris, first of the land, to flourish." And so it went on. After a while he had me finish to his dictation.

When we had done, he picked up another papyrus and read out a recipe for removing wrinkles from the skin. "It's made from the oil of the helbah seed. When you are old," he laughed, "it will keep you attractive to women!" Oh! Seneb you could not know what you were saying.

"But come," he went on, laying down the papyrus, "I have more important work for you." And he reached across the table to push a heap of papyri towards me. "These are for you to copy."

I took them to my table. They were a strange mixture; most were the usual recipes, yet others were quite old and Seneb could throw no light on their origins. But stranger still were their contents which seemed to bear no relationship to their age. As I worked my way through, I saw quite soon that they simply reflected the unchanging state of medical affairs. Herbal remedies in abundance; recipes including milk, honey, the fat of an amazing variety of animals and the salts of many minerals were all intelligently prescribed. Not so welcome were those

---

* This copy is evidently what is now known as the Edwin Smith Papyrus after the man who acquired it at Luxor in 1862. The copy is believed to date from 1600 BC; the translation by James H. Breasted was published in 1930. – J.G.
** The Edwin Smith Papyrus does, in fact, stop in mid-sentence. The incantations on the back, mentioned by Dr Baldassare, are only partly in the same hand, so it would appear that he was responsible for writing the remainder. – J.G.

that had their basis in magic and superstitious beliefs and were intended to repel evil spirits or attract benevolent deities; most revolved around the fluids and organs of the body and the excreta of man and animals, both real and fantastic. Unpleasant and irrational though these were, some of the more outlandishly sounding ingredients were merely secret names given to common herbs in order to preserve the priestly mystique.

One papyrus, however, aroused my curiosity. It was newly written, but whether derived from the writer's own observations or whether copied from another source, I could not discover. It told of the heart's movement and how this could be felt in many parts of the body: "the heart speaks out of the vessels of every limb"*. Imhotep's voice could still be heard even if only in the faintest of echoes.

As I copied on, curiosity gave way to unease. In my innermost heart I knew it was the gods who governed each man's destiny. Yet my continued existence on earth was beginning to persuade me that only in mankind's acceptance of Imhotep's teachings lay the route to my salvation. But alas! these faint echoes had always been swamped by folk medicine and superstition. For all practical purposes, the tangible evidence of his wisdom might have remained buried in the sands of Memphis. I was no nearer extricating myself from my predicament. So, after all these years, I decided the time had at last come for me to seek out new lands.

I left Seneb and without pausing to say goodbye, I travelled by boat down the Nile. Past Enet, Shem, Du-Kau, and Akhetaton. On past Menet Hufu until at length Imhotep's pyramid rose step-wise out of the mist. No longer resting alone in its magnificence, for now those of Khufu, Khafre and Menkaura** and other long-dead kings thrust their threnetic peaks at the sky.

On I went by Tyre and Sidon; and then I came to Byblus.

---

* This is contained in the Ebers Papyrus, obtained at Thebes in 1872 by Georg Ebers and published by him in facsimile in 1875. It is believed to date from about 1500 BC. – J.G.
** Better known by their Greek names of Cheops, Chephren and Mycerinus, respectively. – J.G.

2

Life in conflict with death*

I n Byblus my heart sang.

Long ago, when I was a child, the people of Akkad had not been alone in viewing Nature's moods and seasons in terms of human experience; where else had we to look but at ourselves? We were born; we married; we gave birth and we died – and so, too, did the gods who governed our world. In their anger, they unleashed the wind, the rain, the thunder and the lightning. In their pleasure, they smiled and the sun shone on our fields. The plant spirits of our ancestors were transmuted into the gods of vegetation and were, like ourselves, life in conflict with death. Should they die and not be reborn, we also would suffer and die. So, to ensure their return, we played out the cycle of change in our worship. [You, Dr Annandale, will no doubt see here the origins of homeopathic or imitative magic – like produces like.]

As I had discovered in my wanderings, there were numerous variations about this central theme, but the essence of them all was that the people's corn god had to be killed and descend into the underworld. There, his goddess would follow to strike a bargain with the resident deity that allowed her beloved to return to spend part of the year on earth – and woe betide him if he failed to report back to Hades for the remainder. With the passage of time, the rituals of death and rebirth were united in a single festival that varied only in degrees

*The mythology of the Eastern Mediterranean and the medicine of Babylon. c. 1500 BC. – J.G.

30

of licentiousness and cruelty from age to age and from culture to culture. And, also as time passed, people lost touch with the origins of their devotions and reached the ridiculous situation in which the god became his own enemy and was himself sacrificed to himself. The circumstances in which I reached Byblus accounted for my getting caught up as the lead player in one of these festivals.

*   *   *

The hands that pulled me from the sea were the rough calloused hands of fishermen. My ship had foundered in the last of the winter storms and the mounting agony of those days alone in the sea, when all my companions had perished, gave me further proof, if proof were needed, of the paradox of my mortal immortality.

It was my eyes that once again settled my immediate fate. When I managed to open the painfully swollen lids, I saw the face peering anxiously into mine draw back in wonderment; almost in reverence. The owner of the face lurched to his feet and started muttering to another member of the crew. When I next looked up, I had the distinct impression that my arrival was not unexpected.

"Tammuz." His voice was scarcely audible above the clamour of wind and sea. "Tammuz, you are welcome...." But I heard no more as I vomited horribly and lapsed once again into insensibility. The more unpleasant aspects of the mortality denied me were not to be evaded.

I dreamed that it was the dawn of the first day. A new life was born within me. I was warm and comfortable; my spirit was young again and the languor of sweet content pervaded my whole being. In the distance, women's voices sang to the accompaniment of a solitary flute. Perfume laden with the freshness of spring drifted over me on the faintest of breezes. But reality was not far away; the hands that washed my body with pure fresh water and bathed my sores in scented oil were the soft gentle hands of a mortal creature. I slept again.

When I awoke I was aware, through the mists that shrouded my mind, of another's presence. I felt her fingers touch my cheek, tentatively as if unsure of themselves. Then came certainty, and my face was caressed by those gentle hands; she kissed me. Her lips were balm to mine.

Only once had I known a kiss like this – a kiss of such simple intensity. But then it had been the herald of death. Now it greeted the dawn of a new life.

I remained still, allowing my strength to return. When, at length, I roused myself sufficiently to view my surroundings, she had gone. I was lying on a vast couch and dressed in a robe of softest red linen. One side of the room was a single long opening, broken at intervals by decoratively carved pillars. From where I lay, I saw only the sea beyond, as if from a great height. I turned my head; what I thought to have been a room was but one part of a series of colonnaded cloisters surrounding a marble-tiled courtyard open to the sky. In its very centre, a tall elegant obelisk drew down the warmth of the sun. The atmosphere had the innocence of youth. I continued to lie there absorbing the healing peace.

A movement, caught by the corner of my eye, made me raise my head. She was there after all, studying me from the shadow of one of the pillars. I watched as she walked across and kissed me, this time on the brow.

"Welcome Tammuz!"

"Why do you call me Tammuz? And the fishermen, too? It is not my name. I am called...." But no, I would wait for her answer before telling her.

After a moment's contemplation, as if bewildered by my failure to grasp what was so evident to her, she answered my question.

"In a dream the gods told me that Tammuz would not this year be chosen by the priests; he would be a stranger brought to Byblus by the sea. So, when the priests brought you here, I knew that you were to be my Tammuz."

She bent over and kissed me again. Her long hair, like an autumn sunset, fell across my face. The years were kissed away; the girl who, in a distant bygone age had given her life that the eternal law might be fulfilled, was born again. My arms reached out and drew her down beside me. Gently, she escaped.

"Tammuz, the time is not yet." Her soft low voice was a wind to the flames of my desire. My body called for her. For the first time in my existence I felt, not lust, only a love that dominated every fibre of my being – if this was to be my new life, I would joyously live for ever.

She moved away while I lay back and gazed at her in wonderment.

"Who are you?" I was curious to learn what she believed as I was certain she was ignorant of her role in the eternal game.

She turned; my pulses quickened. "I am...." She stopped and, looking down, began twisting the ends of her sash between her fingers. The tears welled up. "I have no name. As a child I was taken captive and brought to Byblus. Even as a child I was beautiful." She blushed and smiled, but she spoke the truth. "I was raised in the sanctuary of Astarte, the easier for her spirit to become my spirit. You are in my sanctuary now; I am Astarte!"

"Then I shall call you Ishtar," I interrupted. "That is your name in my country. And you shall call me Bal-sarra-uzur, the man who brought you back to life." And for the second time she looked at me in perplexity, but before she could ask what I meant, I started to tremble, cold as I still was from my long battle with the sea. She lay down and drew the cover closely around us.

"Rest, Tammuz, rest." Her voice and the warmth of her body comforted me greatly.

"Why do you still call me Tammuz, when you know my name is Bal-sarra-uzur?" I asked when the spasm had passed.

"Your body may be that of Bal-sarra-uzur, but your spirit is that of Tammuz. To the people of Byblus you are the god risen from the dead to be my lover. I am Astarte and her spirit is within me.

"Each year the chosen one of Astarte journeys into darkness to bring Tammuz back to his people. It is like this: Unless a stranger comes to the city in spring, the most handsome youth assumes the mantle of the god. It is a great and sought-after honour as the sacrifice ensures his immortality." I said nothing, as I did not see this as the ideal moment for questioning the delights of that condition. "If Tammuz is not reborn," she continued, "there will be no lover for Astarte and the harvest will fail. No children will be born and Byblus will fall into decay and ruin. You are my Tammuz!"

Ishtar felt for my hand. "But who are you? You were pulled alive from the sea when any mortal man would have perished."

"My name truly is Bal-sarra-uzur and I come from Babylon in the east," I answered. "I am a physician who travels in search of understanding. In moments of despair I believe my search to be in vain."

I stopped, aghast at what I had just said. The image of Imhotep in his ibis-headed mask came, unbidden, in vivid anger before me; then, as quickly as it had come, it faded.

"No!" I cried, for in that moment I had seen the greater purpose of my search. "No! I have found what I was seeking. It is love. The love of Ishtar; the love that was given me at the beginning of time and shall endure until its end. Love is the source of the understanding that I seek!" I was ecstatic at the revelation. [You, Dr Annandale, will appreciate that, even after a thousand years, my emotional development was still that of a twenty-year-old!]

I was wrong, of course, hopelessly wrong. Maybe one day long years hence...? But at this moment I was happy, truly happy. I now believed that love would free me from the spell Imhotep had cast upon me. Ishtar and Bal-sarra-uzur – Astarte and Tammuz – would walk together, hand-in-hand to the land from which there can be no return.

The day ended and darkness came. The night blessed us with its tranquillity.

In the days that followed, holy rites were celebrated in the courtyard, centred around the obelisk, the image of the goddess. We took no part. Our contribution began one morning when we were summoned early and ordered to leave the sanctuary. Descending a steep twisting stone staircase we took our places in the great procession already forming in the street below. For the whole of the day we journeyed inland climbing steadily, and all the while the flutes wailed and the people chanted a mournful lament, weeping and whipping themselves until their blood laid the dust at their feet.

"Ishtar, why this misery?" It was wrong that others should not be sharing in my happiness.

"Tammuz goes to his death and Astarte to her grief. It is of that they sing. We shall be alone and as surely as winter shall come so must Tammuz die." She looked at me and again there were tears in her eyes.

The next morning I awoke to find it as Ishtar had said. The people of Byblus were gone and we were alone in a small stone temple prepared for our comfort and delight. I went outside into mountain air of inexpressible clarity and sweetness. If I were indeed to die there could be no lovelier place. The temple itself had been built in a cedar grove set in a natural amphitheatre high in the mountain. But high though we were, cliffs rose, precipice upon precipice into the eastern sky. Across the chasm, almost hidden in shadow, a river of crystal water sprang from a mighty fault in the rocks to disappear far below in the mists of the early morning.

I stood entranced, waiting for the sun to clear the cliffs. Goats were bleating as they browsed sure-footed among bushes on the precarious rock face. Wheeling in the sky high, high above, eagles maintained their relentless vigilance for unsuspecting prey; their majestic grace the only disturbing intimation of impending mortality in this earthly paradise.

The sun came to dissolve the mists and I watched the river plunging from pool to pool in a glorious tumble of falls until it again disappeared in a valley of deepening shades of green that carried it at last to the open sea. Butterflies rose in clouds to mate in the warming air, leaving beneath a profusion of sweet-scented flowers.

I was a god in the glory of his dominion.

Ishtar held me from behind. "The waters of the river will soon be dyed with the blood of Tammuz and the anemones will be stained red."

"My love, Tammuz may die but Bal-sarra-uzur shall live for ever with his Ishtar!" At that moment I exalted in my immortality. I turned and crushed her to me, a prayer on my lips that our mortal bodies would unite in that immortality.

"How is Tammuz to die?" I asked.

"He hunts the wild boar, but one day Allatu, jealous of Astarte, breaks his spear on the rocks to leave him defenceless. He is killed by the boar. In due time, Allatu releases Astarte and she is saved by a priest from Byblus."

"Allatu?"

"She is the goddess who rules over the land of the dead."

"Then we are safe, my Ishtar; you are the only goddess who can have power over me." And sitting by her side I told her my story.

When the river below turned blood-red – dyed with red earth as it swept along in its flood – we left the temple by the path to the east. Tammuz was dead, but this year his body would not be found and there would be no Astarte to grieve for him.

*   *   *

The road to Babylon was long. Yet I was irresistibly drawn to the city, perhaps to escape a mythological death but more, I believe, to witness the great changes taking place in the country of my birth. And wherever I chose to go, Ishtar was at my side.

Hammurapi, king of Babylon, an excellent and humane man, had achieved political stability among the petty states of Akkad before conquering Sumer and establishing himself as supreme ruler of

Babylonia. He took an innocent pleasure in referring to himself as King of the Four Quarters of the World. Although the kings of Akkad before him had been the human agents of the gods – unlike the pharaohs who were divine in their own persons – Hammurapi did not assume divinity in any form. Nevertheless, to ensure a favourable reception when the time came, he dedicated his achievements to the gods and had them inscribed on a mighty block of basalt. Some said that these were laws handed down to him by the gods but, as this thoroughly pragmatic monarch remarked, if the people chose to believe this and it made them happy, who was he to disillusion them.

Shortly after leaving Byblus, Ishtar became convinced that Allatu was following us. The Queen of Darkness had been cheated of Tammuz and now, said Ishtar, in her vengeance demanded the soul of Astarte. No amount of reasoning on my part could shake this conviction; the Ishtar at my side was a mortal child of circumstances, not an immortal goddess.

The first proof of what to her was Allatu's wrath came when we reached Kadesh. I had returned from bribing a camel-master to find Ishtar frightened and weeping. With shaking hands she showed me a piece of cloth stained with blood that had risen into her mouth.

"Allatu has come to destroy me. We cannot deny the gods what is rightfully theirs and hope to escape their anger." Her voice was muffled and faint. She coughed and her blood flowed again.

I knelt and took her hands. They were cold. "It will pass," I said with a confidence I was far from feeling. The wings of the little bird of hope fluttered only feebly within my heart: I had seen many die from a simple beginning like this.

Yet pass it did and we set out into the desert. The journey was harsh and even the strongest amongst us suffered. At Derez Zor we boarded a boat to take us down the Euphrates to Babylon. Ishtar was a very sick woman. Her flesh had begun to fall away; she craved for spiced dishes but would not eat, and by nightfall her tiredness was extreme even though she had rested through the day. When I took her in my arms at night, her skin was drenched with sweat and she would start the morning by coughing away the decay that was rotting her body.

Despite her pathetic physical deterioration, all her senses were heightened and she was happy, confident that once we reached Babylon, we would be under the protection of her goddess namesake and all would be well again. There was an unnatural quality about this confidence which disturbed me.

At Babylon, Ishtar was carried ashore on her couch, while I acquired a house and servants and went to seek a physician. In the market place my enquiry was met with the choice between a practitioner of medicine or of magic. My puzzlement was evident.

"You are a stranger here?" I answered that I was newly arrived from Phoenicia and that my wife was wasting away.

The man thought for a while. "You should, I think, discover the divine intentions of this sickness." And he gave me directions to a practitioner of the magic art.

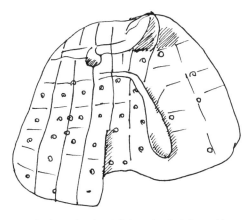

Clay representation of a sheep's liver from Babylon – though similar models were used in other ancient cultures. The liver of the sacrificed animal was carefully compared with the model and the position of any deviation on its surface pegged out in the holes on the clay. The result formed a basis for divining the nature of the patient's disease.

I found the man in a temple where he took my money before bidding me breathe into the nostrils of a sheep. Ishtar should have done this, but when I explained that she was too sick to be moved, he agreed that I, as her husband, would serve as well. He then sacrificed the beast and removed its liver. This, he examined with great care, consulting various charts before giving me a magic formula. It was, need I say, useless for any purpose. Not much had changed since the days of my youth.

Walking away, I heard a voice within my head – perhaps the echo of Imhotep's – insisting: "Find a physician. Find a physician." I obeyed. The man who accompanied me home was clean-shaven and, besides a bag of herbs, carried a libation jar and a censer, the insignia of his calling. As he studied Ishtar, I saw a look of hopelessness momentarily cross his face. Nevertheless, he prescribed a number of herbal concoctions which, he said, would ease the pain of her breathing and help her to rest more peacefully.

When I mentioned that I also was a physician but from a distant land, he was eager to tell me of the reforms introduced by Hammurapi, as he believed these to be unique to Babylonia.

"We have many herbal remedies that banish sickness." [He was correct in this, Dr Annandale, as some of the herbs had medicinal properties that you would recognize today, though others were quite useless. The physician's skill – or luck – lay in prescribing the correct one.] "We physicians are rewarded according to the nature of the sickness and the worth of the sufferer. *Our* worth is judged by what we decide to treat and what we decide to leave to those who rely on magical potions! If we fail to banish the sickness or the sufferer dies, we have a penalty to pay, which likewise depends on the worth of the sick man. Yet we fare better than the surgeons; if they are inept, they are liable to lose their hands. Fortunately, most of their work is setting broken bones and removing the impediment that clouds the sight – and they are skilled at both."

When the physician had left, I returned to Ishtar, the earthly shadow of my Ishtar. Her cheeks were flushed with a hectic fever but from their sunken sockets her eyes blazed with her desperation to live. She struggled for breath while I could only watch her agony.

Then, at the end of a day when the wind had whipped the desert sand into a fury and hidden the sun from view, I sensed her life was finally slipping away. I hurried to her room. Her eyes were shut, but her cracked dry lips were moving. I bent down to listen.

"Allatu has come for me at last. Goodbye, Bal-sarra-uzur, for ever my only love." And there was no stopping her life's blood as it poured from her mouth.

When my tears had ceased, I raised my head from her poor destroyed body. In the shadows – though my whole world was now in shadow – stood a woman. She was tall with only a loose silken cloak to shroud her sensuously dusky skin. Her hair, black as jet, hung thickly in closely curled ringlets to her shoulders. Her lips were full and moist, her nose had the makings of an imperious hook, yet it was her eyes – the darkest of nights in which were reflected the flickering of the lamp like stars at sea – that commanded attention. She surveyed me with contempt.

"Yes, I am Allatu!" she answered my unformed query. "As Babylon weeps for her children with tears that are dry, so shall you weep for Ishtar."

Despite my reluctant acceptance of Imhotep's belief in the natural cause of disease, death remained beyond my comprehension, and with the passing of the centuries I had every justification for my continued belief that it could be nothing other than a divine intervention.

"Ishtar!" As Allatu spat out the name, I saw the spirit of my love rise from the couch and leave with the goddess of the dead.

As they disappeared, I swear I heard Ishtar's voice answer in defiance, "One day the tears of Babylon shall flow again."

3

*Hippocrates describes the doctrine of the four humours**

ar away in the northern sky the storm clouds gathered over Mount Olympus. The purpled edge of darkness hung from the vault of heaven to be rent asunder by brilliant flashes of anger as Zeus hurled his thunderbolts one by one into the earth beneath. Behind the little town of Tricca the hillside lay enveloped in a swirling, eddying curtain of mist. All Thessaly trembled and waited for the god to speak.

The pebbles on the track glistened in opalescent light, as down the centre the mist condensed into human form, attenuated wisps falling away on either side only to roll in again at once as if to mask his progress. The man walked slowly, his head bowed deep in thought. His sandled feet trod with confidence, the weighty staff in his hand more an encumbrance than a help. The robe, gathered over his left shoulder, bared his chest; its hem was wet. At the man's side trotted a short, bare-footed creature shrouded in a hooded cloak. As he drew closer, the man sensed my presence and raised his head. In his clear, wise eyes was recognition.

Puzzled at this, I studied him closely. Yes, there was something familiar about him. Little of his face was visible, hidden as it was by a luxuriant beard shimmering with minute droplets of mist. In my mind's eye I began to picture the face as if shaven. Recognition continued to

---

*Greek mythology, the plague of Athens and the teaching of Hippocrates. c. 1200 BC. – c. 425 BC. – J.G.

elude me until he spoke.

"Surely, Bal-sarra-uzur, you have not forgotten me?"

The emotion that filled my breast was overwhelming. When I had last heard that voice, it had spoken a different tongue but so powerfully did it bring memory flooding back that I lost my hold on the present. The vapours around him assumed unreal shapes. The bare rocks were the pillars of a house; the dusty shrubs, withered in the heat, its richly coloured garden of flowers; the dry bed of the mountain stream bubbled to send its waters springing like fountains into the air. Imhotep stepped from his home and led me into the swirling mist to stand before him in the temple. I heard him speak the fateful question and, in all the vividness it had held for me then, I saw again Ishtar reaching for my kiss, her side gaping from the sword's thrust. I cried out as I crumpled to the ground.

The rocky mountainside returned to its parched reality as, with infinite understanding, Imhotep gave me his hand.

"Imhotep is dead, but his spirit lives on within me. It is Asklepios who speaks with his voice."

Unashamedly, I embraced him, holding tightly until a measure of control had returned. Then, my voice still unsure of itself, I asked, "Master, why are you here? What are you doing? Is Thessaly your new home?" While questions poured from me, the storm drew closer; then in a moment of inspiration, I saw the purpose of our meeting.

"Master, you have come from Zeus with my release. I cannot live for ever!" Desperation overcame me. "If you love me as a son, you will obey the gods and end my agony!" I fell to my knees before him and kissed his hands.

He waited before giving his answer.

"Bal-sarra-uzur, truly I love you, but I no longer have power to change your destiny. My purpose now is to bring the knowledge of Egypt to this land. You should be glad for it will add to man's understanding of disease. The seeds of a new civilization lie here in Greece and when they awaken their glory shall be unsurpassed. But your life, Bal-sarra-uzur, must continue; it is for others yet to come to achieve your salvation. There can be no other road to release!" I am certain I glimpsed a tear in his eye; the depths of my misery were no secret to him.

Together we walked on down the path, the unnatural light casting deep shadows among the rocks. The track was steep and the stones underfoot loose and treacherous. As we crossed the bed of the stream, Asklepios spoke again. "If I cannot bring you rest from this life, I can," he looked at the little figure perched on a rock, "I can give you a companion. Telesphorus is my son; he shall go with you to share your burden and bring strength when your soul is in torment."

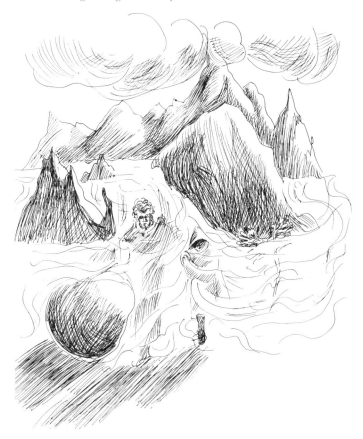

Asklepios and Telesphorus. The mist condensed into human form… at the man's side trotted a short, bare-footed creature shrouded in a hooded cloak.

Telesphorus looked up at me; as he did so the hood fell back. Never had I seen such an impish face. It was the face of a child, a youth, a young man, an old man – it was the face of a being for whom age had no meaning. The expression was full of devilment but quite without malice. His chin was small and pointed; his nose upturned; his eyes were the blue of gentian and tilted imperceptibly upwards at their outer corners; his ears set high and coming to the faintest of points were made to catch the slightest sound; his blond hair lay close to his skull in tight little curls. Immediately, I sensed a bond between us.

"Telesphorus," I said, lingering over the syllables, "will you do as your father says?"

"Yes, Bal-sarra-uzur, I shall do so willingly. You see," he twisted his head to glance at his father, who gave an imperceptible nod, and then turned back to me, "my father has the blood of gods flowing in his veins. So I am immortal and the prospect of accompanying you, even to eternity, holds no terror – in fact, I shall make it a pleasure for both of us." He jumped off the rock, grinned and winked at me.

Great drops of rain now started to fall, marking their arrival with little pits in the dust. Glancing back, I saw Zeus descend from Mount Olympus out of the darkened sky; as his thunderbolts came closer, roars of fury shook the earth.

"Imhotep was mortal," Asklepios said, "but I am truly immortal – Apollo was my father although he entrusted my upbringing to Chiron, the centaur." [At that moment, Dr Annandale, I doubted the truth of his claim as the gods were liberal with the distribution of their seed and no self-respecting family in ancient Greece (and, later, in Rome) was without a god among its ancestors. But I soon realized that, as he said, he was a true immortal.] "So well did Chiron instruct me in the art of healing that Zeus is in a rage." He paused for a moment in contemplation. "It appears that the population of the Underworld is declining and Hades holds me to blame!" His voice smiled at the thought.

"I want you to meet two of my daughters," Asklepios said as we reached the welcome shelter of his home. "They may help you understand man's attitudes to disease." In answer to his call, two exquisitely beautiful girls, dressed simply in white with golden fillets binding their fair hair, appeared from an inner room. There was humanity and compassion in their gaze. But there was something else besides – an impression that their love would never be won by mortal man. They were symbols of what mankind sought on earth, but would, it seemed, attain only in heaven.

Asklepios introduced them to me. Then, reading my thoughts, he went on, "Hygeia and Panacea will always be sought by man – and, as you will discover, he will do so with increasing intensity the more his knowledge expands. Hygeia, he will seek to grant him health throughout his life; Panacea, to cure him of all his ills. In his ignorance, he will confuse the one with the other. And when I am gone, they will take their places on Mount Olympus, for ever inaccessible to earthbound mortals."

At these words, the blackened sky became a moment of purest silver accompanied by a roar that shook the house, reverberating back and forth among the hillsides until its echo faded and died.

"My children," Asklepios rose to his feet, "Zeus demands my life and I must go to meet him. Bal-sarra-uzur, you have my son Telesphorus for company on the road ahead. Though he may not appear so, he is wise and through him you will discover much about the nature of man. Learn and profit."

He bowed his head and remained silent for a while before kissing each of his children in turn. Then, placing Telesphorus's small hand in mine he walked to the door and into the night.

Still grasping Telesphorus by the hand, I followed. The rain had ceased. There was Asklepios, a serpent wound halfway up his staff. Suddenly the heavens split asunder, a tearing blinding flash drowned the darkness and a mighty sound filled the night. Asklepios stood still, gazing upwards, the central point of an ethereal brilliance that dimmed the fury of the thunderbolt.

*   *   *

The relationship between myself and Telesphorus soon developed into one of master and servant – not that I wished it that way, but he was tireless in anticipating my every need and while he was with me I never wanted for food, drink or pleasure. He also appreciated my desire for solitude and from time to time I would awake in the morning to find him gone. Where he went I never knew.

For some while I was deeply troubled by Asklepios's remark about his daughters. To my mind they held the key to man's understanding of disease but now they were gone, leaving behind only confusion. My one hope lay with Telesphorus – who was, after all, their brother. I made the decision to question him one day as we wandered among the wooded hillsides on our way to Athens and had stopped to bathe. The stream bubbled over the rocks with a welcome chill.

"Telesphorus," I said, "if Hygeia and Panacea hold the secret to the understanding of disease, why did they follow Asklepios and abandon mankind to its fate?"

Before answering, he paused to gather his thoughts. Evidently the explanation was not to be simple.

"Mankind has many things to learn, Bal-sarra-uzur," he said, his eyes closed and his normally smooth brow gathered in concentration. "Man cannot expect the gods to lead his life for him – he may look to them for inspiration, but that is all. This may seem hard as life is full of deception. Indeed mankind journeys through life as through mists of illusion. Sometimes the mists part to give glimpses of encouragement before closing again – as you noticed when you first met my father. Men who call upon Hygeia and Panacea, and even on Asklepios himself, for inspiration may be rewarded by a brief parting of the curtain to reveal a fragment of understanding. Those who seek from them a ready answer will find the mist closing more densely around them and will be in danger of losing such understanding as they may already possess."

He smiled and looked at me questioningly. But I said nothing as I believed I had grasped his meaning – and it gave me no encouragement. I saw with an awful clarity that mankind would only slowly, if ever, come to an understanding of disease, keeping me bound to earth for a long, possibly a very long, time.

My thoughts as I plunged into a pool where the icy waters of a small cascade splashed around me, were led back to the origin of my plight. Perhaps the real difference between the beliefs of Imhotep and myself had been one of semantics. After all, if Nature is only another name for the gods, our difference lay in my submission to their will and Imhotep's conviction that he should be able to do something. My difficulty then had been with my belief that, if disease was sent by the gods, it could be anything other than a normal happening. But since Imhotep saw the damage as something that was not normal, he believed it should be possible to help repair the damage caused by Nature.

While lying on the warm, flower-scented ground to dry, I put these thoughts to Telesphorus. His response might give me at least a little encouragement.

"You are right, Bal-sarra-uzur. Both the mortal Imhotep and his immortal Greek manifestation, Asklepios my father, identified the first steps in the understanding of disease."

"Then why," I interrupted more vehemently than I had intended, "why cannot *I* pass on this knowledge?"

"Because no one can give mankind something for which they are not prepared. They would only laugh and hold you up to ridicule. Whenever you are in the company of other people you become as one of them. It cannot be otherwise. Your knowledge becomes no more and no less than theirs. You fall sick and you seek their treatment; you are attacked and you defend yourself with their weapons. Your sole distinction is that you always recover and your wounds heal without trace.

"But do not lose heart. Greece is about to change the world with a glory that shall echo down the centuries. Now, though, I want you to fix your eyes on the greatness of Athens and remember: What is time but another illusion. When, tomorrow, we arrive in Pindar's bright and violet-crowned city, it shall be eight hundred years from today."

*   *   *

In the harsh realities of a city under siege, I would have believed myself free of the world of mythology had it not been for the continued presence of Telesphorus in my life and the perception that ancient myths remain as tributaries of the stream of human consciousness. The evolution of mythology to explain the inexplicable did, after all, reveal an astute insight into the nature of man and an imagination uninhibited by a deeper understanding of the physical world.

[Dr Annandale, I make no apologies for my emphasis on mythology. I can vouch for the fact that the creatures of that world were as alive to the Greeks of some two or three thousand years ago as were the inhabitants of other countries of whom they had only heard tell. The true interpretation of the past is lost with the passing of time, but vestiges of an ancient spirituality lie not far below the surface of any culture – call it part of the race memory if you will. And since much of it has no counterpart today, you find its manifestations inexplicable and perplexing – perhaps even threatening. You must yourself have noticed how the attitudes of some of your patients – and not only the less educated – towards their illnesses, real or imagined, are heavily influenced by considerations of this nature of which they are probably totally unaware.]

Our arrival coincided with the invasion of Attica by the confederacy of Peloponnesian states and to my chagrin we were swept along with the mass of people driven to take refuge in the city. As it was scarcely an auspicious introduction to a glorious new world, I feared Telesphorus had made a serious miscalculation.

"No, Master," he assured me. "This is but a temporary blemish on the face of beauty." I would not myself have described the conditions we met in quite such a romantic manner. Indeed, before long the blemish began to suppurate when the plague, which had come up from Aethiopia through Egypt and Libya, broke out in Piraeus. Rumour had it that the Peloponnesians had poisoned the wells, but when the pestilence spread to the high city it became yet more deadly – and rumour gave way to the fear of uncertainty since the water here was from springs and safe from poisoning. [The nature of the plague, despite Thucydides's excellent description, remains a matter of speculation, as you know, Dr Annandale. I cannot throw any light on it except to suggest that, from what I saw, it might have been a now extinct form of a disease that would be recognizable to you. Alternatively, since it lasted for some five years, it might have been a combination of all the "plagues" that might be expected, given the circumstances. The true interpretation of many past diseases also becomes lost with the passage of time!] Many who attended the sick were themselves quick to die, a point not lost on those self-styled physicians whose interests lay more in the rewards than in the love of their work. They fled the city in unseemly haste at the first opportunity and to no one's great loss: their remedies were as unremarkable in their effectiveness as were all the supplications to the gods or the enquiries of the oracles.

Among the few trained physicians who remained was the Coan, Hippocrates. He came from a family of Asclepiads whose origins could be traced back to Asklepios. [I told you, did I not, Dr Annandale, that a god among one's ancestors was a prerequisite for a good Greek family!] They regarded themselves as highly trained healers and were extremely jealous of their reputation. They lived an itinerant existence visiting villages and towns that were too small to make it worth the while of any physician to settle in the neighbourhood. Hippocrates's fame was widespread, from his birthplace on the island of Cos in the east, through Attica and Thessaly to Thrace in the north. His mere presence at the bedside was reputed to revive the dying. But the charisma of the man was never more evident than in the midst of the moral and physical squalor reigning in Athens. No matter where his patients lay, he was always dressed in clean linen, his hair and beard neatly combed, his nails trimmed and his gentle hands well cared for.

Hippocrates had a vision of medicine which he carried before him all his life. At his home in Cos and on his travels he was constantly teaching, to the extent that at times his everyday conversation seemed to be a series of aphorisms. [Much as the writings of your Mr Shakespeare, Dr Annandale, are full of quotations!] I first met him soon after the outbreak of the plague. He had been up since dawn writing.

"This is the time of the day when I find it most convenient to record my yesterday's observations," he explained after we had exchanged greetings. "I set down every detail, even when events have not gone as I might have hoped. Only in this way will we learn what is normal in nature. I am trying to understand disease by classifying what I observe."

Speculation about disease in general, and its causes in particular, had, he told me, been rife for some while; most importantly, the notion that it was something abnormal had at last been appreciated. [But, Dr Annandale, lacking anything other than the simplest idea of the structure of the body and being in almost total ignorance of how it functioned, the only features of disease that were in the smallest degree comprehensible were those recognizable by one of the five senses. With different diseases having symptoms in common, this led to awesome confusion. Yet it was a start and gave Hippocrates the inspiration to bring order of a sort out of chaos.]

The reason for my visit had been to seek his advice on the treatment of the plague. "State the past, know the present, foretell the future," was his enigmatic reply. "So far as any disease is concerned, strive to help, or at least to do no harm. The art of medicine is threefold: the disease, the patient, the physician. The physician is a labourer for the art."

After a moment's pause, he continued: "Those who make supplication to the gods and enquire of the oracles waste their time. It may well be that the gods rule in heaven and earth, but their influence on our destiny is remote. In medicine natural causes prevail. Diseases are natural events.

"But you asked about the plague. Alas! no physic is of use in these cases. Give barley gruel unless the patient suffers excessively from thirst when water and honey will be best. As to its prognosis, all I can say is that our natures are the physicians of our diseases."

Evidently, he had no better idea than I had. Nevertheless, he was devoting his questioning Greek mind to the problem. Besides grouping illnesses according to their dominant symptoms, he told me he was dividing them into acute and chronic, and into epidemic, endemic and sporadic. As he saw it, until a disease was identifiable as a disease, its cause would remain a mystery and until its cause was known, it could not be adequately treated.

The more Hippocrates talked, the more encouraged I became. His understanding of disease was sufficient to show the way ahead. How I hoped this would satisfy the gods and ensure my release!

I next asked him what he considered to be the cause of the plague. The immediate cause, he said, was the mass of people crowded into the city as this laid them open to attack by an ubiquitous noxious element. What this noxious element was, or where it came from, he was unable to say. And this, regrettably, showed me that any rejoicing on my part would be premature. [The concept of contagion, Dr Annandale, was unknown to Hippocrates, though towards the end of his life there were those such as Isocrates – and later Aristotle – who were convinced that phthisis spread by a corrupt exhalation of the breath. But until the nature of this corruption was known, the concept remained another of the speculations that abounded in medicine.]

"Disease may also come," he continued, "when our digestions are disordered, or from outside sources such as the climate or the geography of the region. If the cause of the disease can be removed, the natural forces within our bodies will overcome the damage it has produced. As physicians, we can help these forces by seeing to the patient's diet and hygiene and the exercise he takes." [How, Dr Annandale, he would have rejoiced when the immune system was discovered.]

When the plague had ceased to ravage Athens, I left the city and journeyed with Hippocrates to his home on Cos. At many places on the way he revealed that, when the occasion demanded, he could be an excellent surgeon as well as the incomparable physician I knew him to be. Among the operations he performed was cutting for stone in the bladder – though this was an undertaking he would only allow trained fellow Asclepiads to perform; no one else should even attempt the operation. The only occasions on which Hippocrates refused to carry out a necessary operation were when he considered the patient might lose too much blood.

For a while I remained on Cos as his guest. My greatest pleasure during these months was to listen while he taught, gathering his pupils under a plane tree. On one of these occasions I learnt about the doctrine of the humours [which, Dr Annandale, was to develop over the ensuing

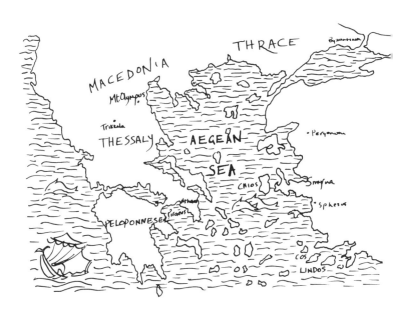

Greece and the Aegean.

centuries and underpin – or haunt, depending on your viewpoint! – medical practice for the next thousand and more years. You will even catch echoes of it in your own time. For the sake of readier comprehension I have taken liberties with his style of speech].

"From the scientific standpoint," he began, "the doctrine of the humours had its origins about a hundred years ago with Pythagoras –

though the medical connection was not immediately made apparent. Pythagoras had spent several years in the temples of Egypt working on a system of numbers that extended back into the astrological recesses of Babylonia and Chaldea. His elucidation of the ancient meaning gave physicians the key to the prognosis of fevers since he believed that certain numbers were endowed with mystic values. On certain days after the onset of a fever, its behaviour determines the prognosis; on certain other days, we know the patient will take a definite turn for the better or the worse.

"But besides working with numbers, Pythagoras challenged the age-old belief that the heart was the seat of life, the soul, the emotions and the intellect; he proposed instead that the mind and the intellect resided in the brain. We have no means of proving his proposition, but his reasoning was persuasive. He also maintained that animals as well as man have a soul and that when the body dies, the soul becomes incarnate again in another body.

"On his return to Crotona, he introduced the doctrine of the four elements – earth, fire, air and water – which, in turn, possessed the qualities of cold, heat, dryness and moisture. These qualities he termed contraries – heat and cold were active contraries; dryness and moisture were passive contraries. Everything in the world consisted, he said, of different mixtures of the four elements.

"This philosophical theory was the inspiration for the idea that the body contained four humours, all of which were to be found in the blood."

At this point he called to one of his assistants and, holding his arm by the wrist, made a swift cut into a vein at the bend of the arm. Another assistant caught the flow of blood in a transparent beaker. At a sign from Hippocrates, he placed the half-filled beaker on a table and bound a towel round the arm.

A far-away look came into Hippocrates's eyes. "Long, long ago in the confused and misty beginnings of their existence on earth our ancestors saw that life ebbed away with the blood flowing from a terrible wound. Blood and life were one and the same to them and now, to our philosophers, blood is become the essential fabric of their theories.

"When you watch the blood in this beaker," he came down to earth again, "you will see the humours appear, though if you had a fever the definition of the changes would be clearer."

As we watched, a layer like a bright red jelly began to form on the surface.

"That," he said, "is blood, the humour."

Next, a transparent yellow fluid seemed to be extruded.

"That is yellow bile."

Left behind was a dark-red jelly from which a pale greeny-white layer finally separated. [I was to learn later, Dr Annandale, that the dark-red jelly was regarded as black bile – thus completing the four humours. Hippocrates did not admit of its existence – most confusing!]

"And that layer," said Hippocrates, "is the humour that is called phlegm. When the blood has come from someone who is ill with a fever, the phlegm may appear more quickly on the surface. Each humour, according to the philosophers, is formed and stored in a different part of the body: blood in the heart; yellow bile in the liver; and phlegm in the brain – a most convenient site!"

[Lest, Dr Annandale, you should find this too fanciful and imaginative, I think I should point out the modern equivalents of the four humours. First, blood when shed is red, then, as coagulation proceeds, serum (the yellow bile of the ancients) is extruded. The dark-red jelly (black bile – which they believed was formed and stored in the spleen) consists of red blood corpuscles enmeshed in fibrin, and phlegm is what you, Dr Annandale, call the buffy coat and consists mainly of white blood cells and platelets. Admittedly, the eye of faith was required as the buffy coat really only appears as such after centrifugation. But if you think about it, the ancients were nearer the truth – as you understand it – than they could possibly have imagined. Apart from the more esoteric changes that take place during disease, one extremely common alteration (in trauma, haemorrhage, infections and many other conditions) is leucocytosis* which shows itself in the increased depth of the buffy coat – and it was excess of phlegm that was blamed for so many diseases.]

"This doctrine of the humours is distorted by some physicians," he spoke with feeling, "who maintain that man is nothing but blood [in the humoral sense]; others that he is only bile; and yet others that he is only phlegm. Each pretends, indeed, that there is a unique substance – chosen at random – which changes its appearance and properties

---

* An increase in the number of circulating white cells in the blood. – J.G.

under the influence of heat or cold, becoming thus pleasant, bitter, black, white, and anything else. This is not so! It is utter stupidity!" His indignation was wonderful to behold!

The following summer Hippocrates announced that he would be returning to Greece and asked whether I would accompany him. When I declined, saying that I had long planned to visit the school at Cnidos on the neighbouring peninsula, he stopped what he was doing and led me by the arm into the shade of the plane tree.

"Have you ever met a physician who was trained at Cnidos, Balthasar?" he asked. (I had learnt the wisdom of adapting my name to suit the locality.)

"No," I replied.

"Then I must warn you against their teachings. The Cnidians think more of the disease than of the patient. They see in every symptom a disease which must be treated. This is wrong; you must look to the good of the whole patient. The nature of the body can be understood only as a whole."

A note, almost of anger, had entered his voice. Many times I had heard him rail against those who, with only limited instruction, practised medicine. But this was the first occasion I had heard him speak so vigorously against a school of physicians.

"Why do you feel so strongly about the Cnidians? Surely theirs is only a different approach to the complexity of disease?"

"That may be so." His tone spoke his true feelings more than the words. "But only by observation and appraisal do we learn how the significance of a symptom can vary according to circumstance. In every patient there is a natural balance which must be sought out and restored by gentle and varied treatment.

"Medicine is an art, and the artist is a man who refuses to put the pleasures of the senses or the comfort of the body before the satisfaction of his artistic sense." I now realized that my questioning had turned his thoughts to ethics, one of his favourite topics. "There are some who call themselves physicians who use their position of trust to debauch the women in the patient's household, who cannot keep the secrets learned at the bedside and who dress and behave in an unbecoming and ostentatious manner. These men do not uphold the dignity of our profession; you should have nothing to do with them." Dear Hippocrates could be rather pompous when the mood took him!

"When you first see a patient, do not discuss your fee," he went on. "If you do, you may lead him to suspect that unless he agrees to your terms you will leave him to his fate. This may be harmful, particularly if the disease is acute. Hold fast to your reputation rather than to profit. It is better to reproach patients you have saved than to upset those who are at death's door."

I left Cos the next day. Hippocrates's parting words to me were: "Love of the art and love of mankind go together." I never saw him again, though his teaching has remained with me and will, I suspect, still be in my heart when I am finally granted peace.

4

*Greek learning is taken to the ends
of the earth by a god in human form**

Hippocrates was correct in his opinion of the Cnidians. Their narrow-minded concept of disease did not, in reality, differ greatly from that of my Akkadian ancestors: both behaved as if disease existed as a thing apart from the body. Since there was nothing for me to learn, I hurriedly took my departure from Cnidos.

When I had been with Hippocrates I had been able to share the clarity of his vision. But on my return to Greece I found that the essence of his understanding of disease was in danger of being drowned in a torrent of medical philosophy. The first signs of this had appeared while Telesphorus and I had been making our journey through time to Athens and, indeed, Hippocrates had approved some of its aspects. But so many physicians and philosophers were now expounding such a variety of theories on the nature of disease that my immediate difficulty was to discern the main stream of thought. My confusion was not eased by the fact that many of these theories were subsequently ascribed to Hippocrates – as were a number of aphorisms that I know were not his. In consequence, my recollection of those times is hazy and I now find it difficult to be precise about the chronology or who said what.

Before moving on I needed, for my own peace of mind, to know whether Hippocrates had really advanced the understanding of disease or whether his work had been without a sure foundation.

*Aristotle and his pupil, Alexander the Great, founder of the most prestigious centre of learning in the ancient world. 370 BC. – 321 BC. – J.G.

"Balthasar," Telesphorus had the voice of one who knew the past but had also visited the future, "Hippocrates stood at the gateway, but the gods denied him admission as he lacked the keys to the doors beyond. Before a physician can understand what is truly abnormal, he must have a complete understanding of what is normal. This was not granted to Hippocrates, although in many instances he did appreciate that what he saw was, in fact, *not* normal." [This may seem self-evident to you, Dr Annandale, but once again you must forget what you know if you wish to reach into the minds of people who lived before your knowledge was acquired.]

"Hippocrates understood that diseases had their patterns," continued Telesphorus. "His attempts to classify them were to enable the same disease to be recognized as such by all physicians. He knew that, if it could be identified, every disease had its cause; but with observation his sole instrument, he could do no more than identify certain responsible conditions. He understood also that treatment could influence and, sometimes, cure a disease – but, more importantly, he knew that the body had the power to recover by itself, unless overcome by the severity of the disease.

"Although his work is treated with disdain by some of the present schools of philosophy, it contains elements of true understanding which will always survive. Even so, for this to happen knowledge of his teachings must be spread throughout the world.

"I know you rarely accept my advice," there was a wicked twinkle in his eye as he said this, "but I think we should journey to Mysia to meet Aristotle, not so much because he is a great and influential philosopher, but for where his friendship will lead."

I asked no questions as Telesphorus would never allow me to base my decisions on a knowledge of future events. We simply made our way across the Aegean Sea to Mysia.

*   *   *

I first met Alexander of Macedon, the last of the gods to walk this earth, when I came to Pella with Aristotle. The philosopher had been summoned by King Philip as tutor to his thirteen-year-old son.

Aristotle had spent much of his youth in Pella when his father was physician to Amyntas II, Philip's father. I like to imagine it was this hereditary influence that added the scientific drive to his philosophical inclination. At any event, after studying under Plato in Athens, he left for the court of Hermeias in Mysia, already believing himself the superior of his dead master. There he stayed for five years during which he described, mostly from his own dissections, nearly five hundred animal inhabitants of the island of Lesbos and the countries around the Aegean Sea.

He was one of the most restless characters I ever encountered; always searching for facts, facts and more facts. Every scrap of information he obtained he fitted into his plan of the animal kingdom – even if some of the facts became a trifle bent in the process. When he had no first-hand knowledge he borrowed the description which, more often than not, had been gleaned from some traveller's fanciful imagination – he was just as gullible as my poor father.

On our arrival in Pella, Aristotle persuaded King Philip to establish a school in an ancient grove of the nymphs. Paths were cut where he might walk while teaching and in the very centre a belvedere was constructed, ostensibly for his rest.

Alexander's fellow pupils were selected personally by Philip from the noblest families in the land. Amongst them were Ptolemy and Hephaestion the tall, dark, curly-headed boy upon whom Alexander came to rely as the only intimate friend in his life. All were to form the Companions of the Grove of the Nymphs, the elite of Alexander's invincible army.

In the belvedere, Aristotle continued his own work.

"There are similarities and differences between the various forms of animal life," he said to me on an afternoon when Alexander and his friends were exercising their horses. "According to these all life is arranged on a ladder of ascending perfection with man standing on the topmost rung. See here!" he commanded and led me to a table where he had displayed a row of hens' eggs with part of their shells removed. "There you have one animal developing from an embryo to its state of perfection. The truth in microcosm illustrates the truth in the macrocosm."

In his excitement, his lisp became more obtrusive; but more distracting was the way he looked at me, not in the eye, but over the top of my forehead. I think he believed the gods came to learn from him and it was to them he was really speaking.

"This egg," he pointed to one on the left, "is three days old. You can just see the first signs of life in that small red pulsating spot. That is the heart."

He went along the row showing me how, as the eggs became older, more of the developing embryo became visible – the body, the head and the enormous eyes.

"Organs appear in order of their importance; the first is the heart – when its motion ceases, death is inevitable. It is the source of the body's innate heat and the seat of sensation and thought. It is home to the soul."

[Here, Dr Annandale, all is not as it might seem to be to modern eyes. Concepts have changed and words have lost their ancient meanings – sometimes beyond recall; in particular, the intellect of today is not the Intellect as it was understood in the distant past. Although it may appear that the ancients (from Pythagoras onwards) were delving into the mysteries of anatomy and physiology, their arguments were, in fact, on a far more esoteric, spiritual plane. For them, the Intellect (by means of which man discerns what lies beyond the earthly plane) resided in the Heart – not the anatomical heart, but the Heart that is the centre of the soul. Thus, the perplexities of the ancients over the location of the Intellect, the Soul and the Heart should not be taken at anatomical face value.]

I looked at him quizzically. He responded to my challenge. "Are you not aware of its action when you experience pleasure or pain?" That, I could not deny.

"But," I asked, "how do you reconcile this with the views of Pythagoras and Hippocrates who maintained that the brain was the seat of the intellect?"

"Who was Pythagoras? Who was Hippocrates?" Sometimes the arrogance of the man was beyond endurance.

"Did they study the animal body as I have done?" he went on, irritated with me for having doubted his word. "No, of course they did not, otherwise they would have found the brain to be without sensation. They were like Plato who concerned himself not with facts but with theory. Balthasar, I have told you before and I tell you again, knowledge must be built on the evidence of a man's senses. They may at times lead him into error, but only by the accumulation of facts can he hope to arrive at the truth.

"No one can doubt the dominance of the heart. Do not my observations tell me that pneuma is responsible for the transmission of both sensation and movement? Does it not convey information from our senses to the heart and is it not the medium through which the expanding and the contracting of the heart bring about movement? Plato refused to trust the evidence of his five senses; he was overwhelmed by his belief that mankind would arrive at the absolute truth through inspiration. But I tell you he was seeking an escape from reality!

"The true duty of the brain, Balthasar, is to cool the innate heat of the body."

Aristotle, by this time, was pacing up and down the belvedere, twisting and untwisting the girdle that held his robe in place, and lisping furiously.

"You see, this is in agreement with my observations that there exist four fundamental qualities, the hot, the cold; the wet, the dry. Each one of these pairs is the opposite of the other. All matter is made up of one from each pair in combination. Thus air is hot and wet; earth is cold and dry. Fire is hot and dry; water is cold and wet. These last two are pertinent to our argument for the fire in the heart must be prevented from overheating the body. This the brain does by secreting a special water we call pituita or phlegm. The lungs help also, by cooling the blood."

I was about to remonstrate with him by pointing out that variations on this theme had been in circulation for many years; that Hippocrates had held rather similar views – which doubtless would have impressed him not at all – when he suddenly stopped his perambulation, looked straight at my forehead and said:

"I have wasted enough time. I am eating with Philip tonight and must change my clothes. Goodbye, Balthasar. You are wiser now than you were two hours ago." And with that his frail, undersized body disappeared through the trees.

Some months later Aristotle introduced into his teaching his beliefs on the soul and on the nature of procreation. Alexander listened with great attention for he was deeply concerned about the mystery of his conception. Philip himself had cast doubts on the legitimacy of his son's birth. His wife, Olympias, the sacred prostitute of Samothrace, had been visited by Zeus in a dream on the night before the wedding ceremony. The lightning of the god had struck fire deep within her womb and the astrologers unhesitatingly interpreted the dream to mean that Zeus and none other had impregnated the beautiful Olympias. By her behaviour and continual worshipping at the altar of Zeus-Ammon*, Olympias did nothing to dispel the rumour. Zeus was the father of her son. [This should not surprise you, Dr Annandale, if you recall what I said about the gods becoming entangled in Greek family trees – and only the greatest of them would suffice for the greatest of earthbound monarchs.]

Aristotle, quite unintentionally, explained for Alexander how this could be.

"Concerning reproduction," he said, "you must understand that the function of the female is to provide the material for the new birth. It is the function of the male to provide the soul, the principle of life. You may view the female part, the material, as the unformed clay to which the hands of the potter give form. The potter contributes nothing material. Thus, since the semen of the male is an accidental and not an essential, it is possible for the principle of life to enter the womb without physical contact."**

A strange look of exultation came into Alexander's face. He continued walking by Aristotle's side, but his thoughts were far away.

Aristotle, seemingly unaware that his pupil was no longer listening, continued: "You may distinguish that which has life from that which has not by the presence of this soul, or psyche, which gives form and leads to the development of perfection. The soul in man has three parts: the vegetative which is concerned with nourishment and reproduction; the animal, which is sensitive; and the rational which is intellectual. The lowest of these is the vegetative; the highest, the rational. Plato would have had us believe that the intellectual or emotional soul was immortal. In his ignorance he failed to relate theory to observed fact and held firmly to what he *wished* to believe." The contempt for his old master's opinion was awesome.

"From what I have said, you can see why love appears in different guises. The love determined by the vegetative soul drives a man to reproduce himself; it is crude and vulgar. The love which a man can

---

* The ancient Egyptian ram-headed god, Ammon, was identified by the Greeks with Zeus. – J.G.
** This deeply philosophical sentence is, strangely, not enlarged upon by Dr Baldassare in one of his asides to David Annandale. To oversimplify matters, it is a statement of the possibility of virgin birth (the offspring being the incarnation of divine powers), belief in which is as old as religion itself. For Alexander, it was confirmation that he was indeed the son of Zeus-Ammon. – J.G

experience through the rational soul transcends the needs of the body; it can be felt by a man for a man; it opens the way to a state of greater understanding." Alexander exchanged glances with Hephaestion; they put their arms around each other's waists. "Thus the female with her defective soul," continued Aristotle, aware of the effect of his words, "is imprisoned within her material body; only a man is capable of transcending all intellectual and spiritual limitations."

I stopped. Aristotle's pupils walked on past me. His words had struck a response deep within me, although I could not define its nature. From my first sight of Alexander I had felt that our destinies were linked. This was a matter I had to discuss with Telesphorus. I made my way home to be greeted by squeals of delight from his room. He was up to his usual tricks and was entertaining one of the girls from the gynaeceum. I banged on the door.

"Telesphorus! I wish to speak with you." I didn't wait to hear his reply.

In what was, for him, a reasonably short time he joined me on the porch. I told him what Aristotle had said and then asked him why I should have felt that the words held a personal significance for me in relation to Alexander.

"The reason, Balthasar," he answered, "is that so far in your long life you have experienced only physical love or, as Aristotle might put it, only your vegetative soul has been aroused. Although ordinary mortals all possess a rational soul, this has to pass through many incarnations before it reaches maturity. Yours, although still in an adolescent state will be put to the test through Alexander."

I pressed him to tell me more, but he refused and with ill grace I allowed him to return to his pleasures. What sort of a soul did he have, I wondered.

Alexander was twenty-one when he left Pella at the head of thirty thousand infantry and seven thousand cavalry to conquer the world.

* * *

The lands of Ammon were under the heel of the foreign invader; in Egypt the Ram-headed god of the Hidden Sun had been defiled by the Persian conqueror. Alexander, the chosen one of Ammon, would restore for the last time the true religion. This was written in his stars, and in mine it was written that I should follow his destiny to the end.

He was received with rejoicing in the city of Jerusalem where his coming had been foretold by the prophet Daniel. And in Egypt he was crowned Pharaoh in Memphis with all the mystic circumstance known to that ancient people. My fellow Companions believed I was overcome by the spiritual glory of the occasion, but the tears I shed were the outward sign of my own tormented emotions. Memphis had more significance for me than ever it would for its latest pharaoh. My first memory of Ishtar would be with me always.

Shortly after the ceremony, Alexander marched with a small body of troops down the western side of the Nile delta until, at Rakoti on the shores of the Internal Sea, he founded the first and greatest of the cities that would bear his name.

The plans were drawn up under his guidance and the sites of all the buildings marked out on the ground: Where the temples would rise to the glory of Ammon, sacrifices were offered and a papyrus was unrolled in symbolic gesture where the library would preserve the written knowledge of the world.

Leaving the work in the capable hands of Dinocrates, his architect, Alexander set out on a spiritual pilgrimage. With only the Companions (amongst whom I had been numbered from the start) to guard him he marched westwards along the coast before turning south into the deserts of Libya. Ten days later, we emerged from a sandstorm to see lying before us the holy oasis of Siwa. As one man we halted and gazed with inflamed, sunscorched eyes at its sheer, utter luxuriant beauty. Here, indeed, was the heart of Ammon; his temples shaded from the glare by groves of leafy palms and olive trees. After the days of hardship in the desert every one of us was acutely receptive to the spirituality of Siwa.

On the steps of the greatest temple the high priest, speaking in Greek, bade Alexander welcome as the son of Ammon. As he finished, the image of the god, preceded by two sacred virgins, naked and accompanying their dance on flutes, emerged from the darkness of the building.

Lying in its wooden coffer, the image was borne by handmaidens of the temple. As they swayed and staggered in the ecstasy of their task, ornaments suspended from the litter created the music of a tinkling bell. The movements and sounds were interpreted by the high priest in answer to whatever question was asked of the oracle.

The Companions were assured that their fortune lay with Alexander and, for some, great wealth and power were foretold. When the image passed before me I asked, quite simply, but in the ancient tongue:

"When shall I die?"

At that moment one of the handmaidens fell senseless to the ground, the ark lurched and nearly slipped from the litter. The high priest paled, but otherwise maintained his outward calm. He looked straight at me.

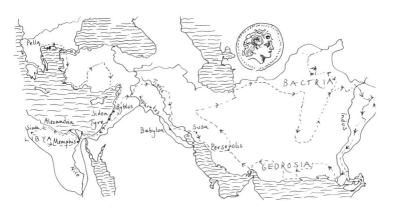

Alexander the Great and his Empire. His march of liberation and conquest is indicated by the broken line.

"Balthasar," he said, and there was compassion in his voice, "it is written that when the light replaces the dark to the uttermost ends of the earth, then shall you die. The nights are many but the god shall be with you always to guard you."

Ptolemy, who was standing beside me, could hardly contain his excitement.

"That was the confirmation of all our hopes," he burst out in enthusiasm. "Alexander shall conquer the world and bring the light of Ammon to all foreign lands, and if you are to live until this is accomplished, so must he, as he is to be your protector."

Alas! I could not share his joy. I knew the true meaning of the oracle's pronouncement. But Ptolemy did not wait for enlightenment and moved away to spread the false interpretation among the Companions. Nor had he noticed the high priest's use of my name; I would have found explanation difficult.

Meanwhile the high priest had returned to the temple taking Alexander with him. What mystic ceremony took place inside, no man shall ever know.

*   *   *

In Babylon, Alexander was feted. He had fulfilled the prophesies and released the lands of Ammon from bondage. The armies of Darius III, King of Persia, had been outmanoeuvred and then defeated.

As we approached the city I became aware of tension mounting within me. I knew, intuitively, that Ishtar was once again living on earth and that I was drawing near to her. I began by studying the faces of all the women I passed, even though I knew this to be useless – long since in my dreams she had ceased to be a remembered figure and had instead become an intense emotion. The living Ishtar would be found when I least expected her. To gain some release from my thoughts, I gave myself to pleasure. I attended banquets without number in honour of Alexander and his generals. We were waited on by the wives and daughters of the highest officials – at the start, they were dressed in the full splendour of their fashion but as the meal progressed they gradually removed their garments until at the last course they were completely naked. Thus did they give thanks to Alexander. I declined to take advantage of their gratitude, preferring instead the oblivion offered by Dionysus.

Whether Alexander was militarily correct to pursue the person of Darius is not for me to judge. Perhaps he was, as the continued presence of the defeated monarch was a threat to the security of his new empire. But this I do know: from the moment that Alexander set out from Babylon in pursuit and left behind the lands of Ammon, he ceased to be a god and became a cruel, brutal conqueror. At times his actions were tinged with madness. The gods were done with him and he was treading with increasing swiftness the path to his inevitable destruction.

*   *   *

Darius was murdered by Bessus, his own cousin. Bessus was betrayed by Spitamenes, his own general, and delivered into Alexander's hands. Spitamenes was slaughtered by his own wife, who came to Alexander carrying her husband's head. But still Alexander strode like an avenging Achilles through the Persian empire. His troops suffered in full measure from the harshness of the climate and the countryside, and only the force of his personality supported by not a few murders of friends both good and bad, enabled him to stave off mutiny.

*   *   *

One prince of Bactria remained unsubdued. From his impregnable mountain fortress, Oxyartes refused to acknowledge Alexander. He considered himself safe since the walls of his stronghold rose in continuation of the precipice at whose foot we were encamped. When Alexander demanded his surrender, Oxyartes replied that only if Alexander's men grew the wings of eagles could they take the fortress.

The following night was bitterly cold and a snowstorm raged with blinding fury. Some time before midnight I had fallen into troubled sleep. Whether I awoke from a dream or whether waking I had a vision, I cannot say, but there standing before me was Ishtar. She was real, vivid and alive; substance impressed itself on emotion and I could see every detail of her beloved face as if the day had dawned. Into my memory flooded the scent of her presence.

She walked towards me, knelt down, took my hands in hers and kissed me on the lips. "Bal-sarra-uzur."

I tightened my grip and responded to the softness of her kiss. Instantly she was gone!

I awoke Telesphorus, who had never left my side since our departure from Pella.

"Telesphorus, we shall be the first of Alexander's soldiers to grow wings. Before dawn I mean to be inside that fortress!"

Surprisingly there was no argument. All he said was, "Then we must hurry." In the darkness we bound skins about our legs and arms and wrapped ourselves in layers of clothing. Telesphorus stuck a knife in his belt; I was unarmed.

The wind was biting; the snow, still falling heavily, covered our tracks as soon as we lifted our feet. We were swallowed instantly by the wilderness of the dark and no one saw us leave.

For what seemed an age Telesphorus led me on. The ground sloped steeply upwards, but there was no sign of the vertical wall I knew we had to climb.

"The snow is stopping, Balthasar," he whispered. "We must take care we are not seen."

A few paces on he came to a halt. "Master, look into my eyes and believe you are standing on the ramparts of Oxyartes's fortress." I did as he said. "All things are possible if your belief is strong enough. Now close your eyes."

I waited. "Balthasar," he spoke close to my ear, "you may open your eyes again. I have led you far enough. You must go on alone, my divinity would only be an embarrassment to you." He laughed softly. "I return to tell the king that one of his subjects has the wings of an eagle and that where one has gone, the rest may follow." And he disappeared over the ramparts*.

I moved cautiously down to the roadway. As there was no sign that I had been seen, I took shelter under an arch to await the coming of dawn. For the first time since leaving Alexander's camp I wondered what I really hoped to achieve. Here I was, alone in a hostile fortress, driven by an ancient passion flaming inside me. Alexander's madness had communicated itself to me.

The new day began. I got to my feet; fate should take a hand in the moulding of events. Slowly I walked on until I came to the gates of the citadel. There was no turning to left or to right. Behind, the approach of marching feet. In front, the closed gates with the guards before them.

Half conscious, cut and bleeding, my clothes all but torn from me, I was dragged into the great hall of Oxyartes and thrown at his feet. The captain of the guard kicked me with pleasure.

"Noble Oxyartes. This man from Alexander's army climbed the walls during the night. We found him outside the citadel."

"Was he alone?"

"Yes, Sire. But I have ordered a search."

"And Alexander's camp?"

"Silent, Sire. No sign of activity."

I looked about me. The hall was low roofed, the furniture stark and simple, yet the walls were hung with the richest of silken draperies, delicately coloured and patterned. The decorations would have provided an emperor's ransom.

My eyes turned towards Oxyartes, seated on his chair of state.

I cried out, a long-drawn cry of ecstasy. Behind him, in all her exquisite beauty, stood Ishtar.

I swooned into deep unconsciousness.

---

* A similar happening brought an end to the siege of Sardis when Cyrus the Persian took the city of Croesus the Lydian, c. 546 BC. (Herodotus, *The Histories*, I, 84.) – J.G.

For days I ran a high fever. When I emerged from my delirium Alexander was standing beside me. With the gentle manner, now so rarely seen, he gripped my hand.

"Balthasar, most noble of all physicians. Welcome back to us. I feared your example to my soldiers had caused your death."

I raised my head. I was lying in Alexander's own tent.

"Tell me how I was saved. Where is Ishtar?" In my weakness I could say no more; yet there was so much I needed to know.

"When your servant returned I had him lead others after you. At daybreak three hundred men were ready to storm the ramparts. They had not been discovered and met with little resistance. Oxyartes is my prisoner."

"Where is Ishtar? Where is Ishtar?" I was insistent.

Alexander gave Hephaestion a puzzled look. "He is raving again," said Hephaestion. "It is better to leave him in Roxana's care."

I lay back exhausted, too weak to plead with them. A cool hand was laid on my brow; I could feel the strength flowing into me. Was I again in Byblus? I opened my eyes. Seated at the bedside was Ishtar. I began to tremble uncontrollably.

"I am Roxana," she said, "daughter of Oxyartes and now wife to Alexander. He has put you in my charge until you are healed."

My brain was in tumult. Her words were spoken as if to a stranger.

"Ishtar, my love, do you not recognize me? Is it nothing to you that we are together again? I am Bal-sarra-uzur. Do you not remember? You have come back to me. Ishtar, love me again!"

"Poor Balthasar." There was tenderness in her voice and her eyes were filled with pity. "I love Alexander. You and I have never met before. I saw you for the first time when you were brought before my father." She might have been talking to a child that had lost its mother.

Then indeed did I realize how terrible was the blow dealt to me by fate.

As the years passed, Alexander journeyed on, consumed by the inner fire of his ambition. Roxana loved him greatly, but I sometimes wondered how much this love was for the man and how much for the temporal power and glory he reflected. As if to soothe my anguish, a strong spiritual bond developed between us and I was never far from her side. Gradually I came to appreciate the noble, self-sacrificing quality that can exist in a love from which all physical passion is divorced.

Throughout the march back from the Indus, across the desert of Gedrosia, which no army had crossed before, through ravaged, burned Persepolis, through Susa and on to Babylon I watched over her. After Alexander's death in the palace of Hammurapi, I grew anxious for her safety. No sooner was his life extinct than his empire was disputed and heads began to fall. The moment Roxana was fit to travel after giving birth to Alexander's son, we fled to Greece.

One morning I awoke to the most terrible commotion. Quicker than light I was in her room, but too late. She was already dying from the assassin's sword thrust in her breast. Her son's body lay cradled and bloody in her arms.

I bent over and kissed her. "Ishtar."

"Bal-sarra-uzur. We meet, my love, at last." Did I really hear those final words or did they arise from the depths of my longing?

5

Ancient concepts of physiology cannot explain the nature of disease *

I n the wake of Alexander's army, and at his express command, came scientists, philosophers, physicians, artists, sculptors, writers, astronomers, all bearing with them the seeds of learning that they might disseminate them throughout the world to testify to the greatness of Greece and of Alexander. The heart of this intellectual empire was Alexandria in Egypt. Its influence would remain undimmed for close on a thousand years.

After Roxana's death, Telesphorus and I made our way to the oasis at Siwa. There, in the sanctuary of the great temple, my spiritual wounds were healed. To add to the poignancy of my loss, I recalled something Telesphorus had said a very long time ago as we lay in a Grecian meadow. "You have been given the power to recognize your love when she returns. You will always find her." But to discover that *she* might not find *me* – if, in truth, she had – until death had claimed her once again was almost more than I could bear.

When I resumed the burden of my life it seemed appropriate that I should visit Alexandria. There, in Ptolemy's museum, I rubbed shoulders with philosophers and scientists from the far corners of the earth. The confusion inspired by the diversity of their opinions led of necessity to compromise – except among the physicians. They argued, and the more they argued, the further did their views diverge.

This, it is not to be wondered at, had the effect of making medicine

---

*The confusion that is Greek medical philosophy deepens. 321 BC. – 30 BC. – J.G.

one of the most popular subjects, for the Greek mentality rejoiced in endless argument. Because of their profound respect for the human body, the Greeks, anatomically speaking, were disinclined to lift even a solitary finger to uncover what they could not see. The Alexandrians – and those who were not Greeks behaved like Greeks – gave their imaginations free rein to explain these unseen mysteries. And should anyone lift that practical finger, the results were trimmed to fit their own particular theory. For these philosophers, disputation was more important than experience; the human mind alone was noble enough to seek out the truth.

Nevertheless, two men gave me cause to hope. Both Herophilus and Erasistratus were intent on expanding knowledge through observation and experimentation; for them, there was more to anatomy than the display of naked bodies at athletic contests.

I had no difficulty in finding Herophilus. He was dissecting the body of a man who had been executed for the murder of his wife – confined within walls, the stench was already worse by far than that of any day-old battlefield. Herophilus's demonstrations were necessarily few, but always popular despite the assault on the senses, as dissections of the human body were a novelty and, once the initial distaste had been overcome, excited immense curiosity. Among the onlookers was Erasistratus.

While Herophilus displayed the convolutions of the brain and distinguished the two major parts of the organ, Erasistratus held his peace. But when the anatomist moved down the table and opened the belly, Erasistratus began to breathe more deeply and run his fingers through his beard. This was the moment he had been waiting for. The structure of the body was unchallengable and there for all to see, but the functions of its various parts were speculative and Erasistratus believed himself to be on safe ground as he had experimented on live criminals condemned to death. [This, Dr Annandale, has always been open to doubt as neither man left any written account of his work. I was never witness to a live dissection, but I have no reason to doubt its veracity.]

Herophilus removed the liver and put it on one side. He then turned his attention to the stomach and duodenum.

"When food has been eaten," he declaimed, "it enters into the stomach where it undergoes coction. This means that the food is triturated, dissolved, heated and fermented. It then is in a semi-fluid state and passes out of the stomach to be taken up by the body."

"Herophilus," boomed Erasistratus. All eyes turned to him. "How do you know this?"

"Hippocrates stated it was so, and...."

"Ha! Hippocrates said so! And you seriously expect us to believe that just because a flatulent old man said it was so, it is so? Why, it is nothing more than a cookery lesson!"

Erasistratus was getting into his stride. Most of the onlookers were becoming bored with Herophilus's pedantic and long-winded commentary and were ready for an argument. It was part of the expected entertainment.

"I was born on Chios and was taught by Chrysippus on Cnidos. And where did *he*," pointing an accusing finger at Herophilus, "learn his medicine?" The sneer with which the word medicine emerged had been well rehearsed. "I will tell you. On the island of Cos. Herophilus is the imitative ape of Hippocrates. At Cnidos I learnt the true medicine."

The conflict between the two men seemed incapable of resolution. Whatever Herophilus stated, Erasistratus went to great lengths to challenge. Nevertheless, I believe their animosity was the driving force behind their achievements.

"I do not form my opinions from what others have done, but on what I myself have done." Erasistratus thumped the table and glared around the room, daring anyone to contradict him. No one did. "In my experiments," he went on, "I have shown that the stomach, by its movements, breaks up the food into a multitude of small particles. These constitute the chyle. The chyle is of two parts. The first contains the elements of bile and is carried to the gall bladder. The second contains the elements of blood and is carried to the vena cava. Dispute that if you can, Herophilus!"

Herophilus knew he was no match in public debate for the bombastic younger man; but however much Erasistratus annoyed him, he was prepared to make allowances since he appreciated that, in their different ways, both were working towards the same ends. Ignoring the tirade, he proceeded with his dissection. Suddenly he looked up.

"Erasistratus," he said with a sparkle in his eye. "You do sometimes agree with me and even make use of my studies when it suits you? No! do not deny it. You know my work on the pulse, of its variations in rate and rhythm in certain circumstances. And you agree with it?"

"Yes." Erasistratus was grudging with his acknowledgment.

"And as there is another point on which we agree," Herophilus continued, "would you explain the function of respiration while I expose the lungs?"

In a less belligerent tone than before, but with evident ill-nature, Erasistratus began.

"We owe the fact of life to pneuma, that most subtle vapour which pervades our whole being. The air we breathe enters our lungs and from there is taken to the heart which contracts and dilates in response to a force inherent within it. In the heart the air is changed into pneuma, our vital spirit, which is then carried to all parts of the body by the arteries. That part of the pneuma which reaches the cavities of the brain undergoes a further alteration into animal spirit for dispersal to the different structures of the body through the nerves, which are hollow. When we make a movement we do so because our muscles shorten by becoming distended with animal spirit." [This concept, Dr Annandale, is not so ridiculous or far-fetched as it might seem if you consider that the "muscles" of some robots in your electronic age are powered by compressed air conveyed to them along tubes.]

"Further, the blood in our body is contained within the veins, at the ends of which are innumerable invisible communications with the arteries. When an artery is cut, the pneuma first escapes; then the blood from the veins and heart is able to flow through these communications and also escape." [Dr Annandale, you cannot help but see how perceptive the ancients were in their gropings towards the truth. Erasistratus realized that the capillaries must exist some two thousand years before they were seen under the microscope. His error in believing that the arteries contained pneuma which had to escape before the blood could flow from an artery is attributable to his intellectual honesty, as he had never seen a corpse whose arteries had bled when cut.]

"But when we come to consider disease, I utterly reject the belief that it is due to disorder of some hypothetical humour, as propounded by Hippocrates and his ignorant followers." Not for long could Erasistratus refrain from disparaging the Hippocratic method. "Fundamentally, disease is due to plethora. There is too much blood and starvation is the treatment."

Herophilus had reached the limit of his patience. "If that is your belief, you are a greater fool than I took you for. If the diseased body contains an excess of blood, the treatment is to bleed the patient. But you refuse to do so because that is Hippocratic practice!" With that he slammed his knife on the table and stormed into his inner room.

*   *   *

The emergence of the new civilization in Greece that Asklepios had foretold had been more in the nature of an eruption than an evolution. Where it had originated remained a mystery and I often thought that Imhotep's answer to my question of where he had gained his knowledge was as applicable to the Greeks as it had been to him. Thanks to Telesphorus I had seen the eruption in medicine at its magnificent best, but I was also witness to its inevitable petrifaction in the stream of philosophical lava that flowed from the initial explosion. Herophilus and Erasistratus had been the last to escape.

In the final analysis philosophers are in the enviable position of being able to talk arrant nonsense and yet be listened to with respect by others who believe they are expounding a profound truth. (Cicero was of much the same mind when he wrote: "Nihil tam absurde dici potest quod non dicatur ab aliquo philosophorum"!) Eventually, when I had suffered from nearly two-hundred years of absurdities, I decided that enough was enough.

"Telesphorus," – who else could I consult? "Telesphorus, explain what is happening. I have listened and tried to understand, but these interminable arguments about animal spirits and vital spirits, about pneuma and humours make no sense. Far from leading to a greater understanding, they are destroying Hippocrates's teachings. If physicians cannot build on sure foundations already in place, what hope is there for me?" Despondency had become a continuous burden: I could see no end to my earthly existence and my heart was aching; despite Telesphorus's company, I felt terribly alone.

"Bal-sarra-uzur." Whenever I was seriously troubled, Telesphorus would revert to calling me by my original name. "I regret that most of what you hear makes sense only to the speaker. Our philosopher-physicians are shut away in their Alexandrian towers – which is just as well for the rest of humanity."

I could not argue with that. The generality of mankind was as well, or as ill, served as it ever had been by herbalists and itinerant physicians and surgeons.

"Once again, we should undertake a journey with deliberate intent – this time to seek enlightenment. I believe Themison to be the one man capable of pulling together the tangled threads of Greek medical speculation."

And so it was that we made our way to Laodicea where the road to the west divides, one fork taking the traveller towards Ephesus and the other, the more northerly, to Smyrna.

Themison proved to be a kindly man of middle years who made us welcome. When he began to talk, however, I feared I was about to be subjected to yet another one-sided theoretical diatribe.

"The body is composed of an infinity of minute particles. I claim no credit for this discovery; it was first proposed nearly four hundred years ago by Democritus and then Erasistratus gave it his approval. Nevertheless, contrary to the belief of those who maintain that there are four elements, these particles are all of a similar nature – but I see you knew this." Although he gave me a curious look, far from being offended, he seemed pleased to have an audience prepared to listen intelligently.

"My contribution has been to explain how these solid, atomic particles may be responsible for disease. They may become too tightly packed, too loosely packed, or too tightly in one part of the body and too loosely in another. The simplicity of this indicates how we should choose our treatment. In the first case, we produce relaxation by blood-letting, purgation and fomentations. In the second, we administer astringents – cold baths, alum, vinegar. In the third – ah! the third is the challenge to the physician as he must do whatever he thinks to be necessary."

He was not at all put out by this lame ending; indeed he regarded it as the quality that gave the essential twist of complexity to ensure that when other less worthy theories had been long forgotten, his would endure.

At this point, Themison rose and crossed the room to remove the top of a lamp. This was in the form of a flat decorated plate with a hole in its centre.

"You must have realized, Balthasar, that my philosophy as a Methodist is Epicurean and can never be acceptable to the Stoics. Consequently they have devised a theory that is as different from mine as it is possible to get." He held up the lamp top. "It is as if *our* medicine is the solid plate, while the Stoics build their medical philosophy on the centre hole!" His face began to crease until, unable to contain himself any longer, he gave way to sobs of laughter.

It was a merry sound and I must admit that the thought of the Stoic physicians contemplating nothingness appealed to my sense of the absurd and I, too, began to laugh. Nevertheless, Themison was showing me, quite unintentionally, how great was the gulf that divided the different schools of medical philosophy. Insofar as the hole in the top of the lamp served to control the flame, so was that nothingness – the pneuma – held to have perfectly reasonable functions to perform. By formalizing themselves into distinct schools, physicians were successfully restricting their freedom of thought. When Themison had dried his eyes on the sleeve of his robe, he continued with his exposition.

"The Pneumatists, as we call them, have quite lost their way. They call upon their recollections of Pythagoras and Aristotle and now maintain that too much heat causes the pneuma to expand and to move more rapidly in the body so that the person becomes excited. Too much cold causes it to contract and move more slowly: the person becomes sluggish. Excess of heat and dryness produces acute diseases and excess of cold and moisture leads to chronic diseases."

When Themison saw that I was about to question him, he held up his hand and continued.

"I have still to mention two other schools of medical philosophy, if only on account of the numbers of their adherents. There are the Empiricists who say: 'The patient is ill. Use your own experience or what you have learnt from the experience of others to treat his complaints and do not concern yourself with the whys and wherefors.' They reject the need for dissection as they say you only see what is dead and learn nothing about the living! And there are the Dogmatists who take the Hippocratic stand that disease is caused by a lack of balance in the bodily humours but have carried it to such extremes that it now defies recognition."

He sat back in his chair and, clearly satisfied with himself, banged on a table and summoned refreshments.

"The originating force behind all our theories," he began again, "is the doctrine of the four humours – though, I admit, many philosophers have, over the years, not been struck squarely by its impact and have been sent spinning away at a tangent. One of their greatest difficulties has been to account for the warmth of the body.

"Pythagoras's theory of the four elements tells us that heat is associated with perfection and strength, and cold with things undeveloped," he explained. "This is why, a short while after Pythagoras's death, Empedocles, in one of his moments of poetic inspiration, concluded that the source of innate heat – of life itself – was the blood.

"Next the philosophers reasoned that innate heat must require cooling and this, they maintained, was achieved by the pneuma inhaled during respiration. After all, Balthasar, they had to find a purpose for respiration, particularly as Aristotle had said that Nature did nothing in vain. However, they extended the function of the pneuma by saying that it was carried to the brain where it was responsible for producing thought and the movements of the body. When pneuma is prevented from reaching the brain, we lose consciousness." [Change pneuma to oxygen, Dr Annandale, and think of the implications.]

"Eventually, the philosophers brought together all the theories and observations at their disposal, and saw how they could help Nature. They believed that phlegm was responsible for most diseases and, being stored in the brain, was ideally situated to pour down and drown the organs beneath – onto the lungs to cause consumption; into the abdomen to cause dropsy; into the bowels to cause dysentery; and into the rectum to produce haemorrhoids. Nature attempts to deal with this, they said, either by losing the phlegm through the nostrils or by drying up the excess with fever. If the excess is not drained and reaches other parts of the body it produces inflammation or leads to abscesses.

"At this point the philosopher-physicians excelled themselves. Phlegm was a humour contained in the blood and was increased in disease. Why not give Nature a helping hand by removing blood from the patient? That, Balthasar, is why blood-letting is now an integral part of the doctrine of the four humours and is regarded as the best means of removing diseased material from the body!

"As time went on, the physicians discovered that an imbalance between the humours could also be rectified by purging, enemas, hot and cold baths, creating issues to promote the flow of phlegm [pus] and much else, usually unpleasant, besides."

Suddenly, Themison stopped. "I sense you are not what you seem."

He looked searchingly into my eyes as if seeking an answer to his uncertainty; not finding it, he shook his head in disappointment and, since he showed no inclination to continue talking, Telesphorus and I made our departure.

[If, Dr Annandale, you think my account of the Greek period unnecessarily confusing and at odds with itself, then, believe you me, you should have lived through it!* Nevertheless, the persistence of the doctrine of the four humours until displaced by your modern scientific approach was no mean achievement.]

* It actually got much worse before it got better! – J.G.

6

The Illustrious Galen, greatest physician in all Rome...*

elesphorus had many talents, yet the one I prized most highly was his ability to dissolve time. As I lived through the days of my life, I experienced the moments as other men did, but when they had passed they contracted into what they really were: insignificant fragments lost in the universe.

When a man is immortal (a fate to which I was now resigned) it is easy for him to acquire wealth – and as easy to lose it. Beautiful women laid priceless jewels on my pillow in vain attempts to learn the secrets I had gathered along my way. Rich men filled my pockets with gold in return for advice – advice which, as often as not, was simple common sense. I had long learnt the transience of material things although I could appreciate their value to ordinary mortals. But since death eluded me, I longed for somewhere that was home; a home to which I could return when I grew tired to find familiar things unchanged and a welcoming face to greet me. Alas! it was not to be, and all my wealth could not make it so.

Even hope seemed denied me. In my worst moments I felt myself no nearer release from life than the day Imhotep had granted a foolish young man his choice. The more I saw of medicine, the more I felt the gods must be playing tricks on me, using me for their amusement. I was returning to my conviction that the beliefs of my childhood were true – or at least as true as we would ever know in this life – and that

*Medicine during the Roman Empire. 166 – 169. – J.G.

some divinity did indeed govern our fate. An appeal to the gods was still as effective – or as futile – as any bleedings, purgings, or enemas devised by man.

One day, Telesphorus took it into his head that the time had come when I should visit Rome. The reason he gave was that "Romans" now inhabited the far corners of the known world and Rome itself was master of a vast empire – though, as he said, not without a certain difficulty in places.

For some two or three hundred years Rome had been the flame around which the moths of Greek medicine had fluttered. They had no opposition in establishing themselves, despite the bad name they earned, as the Romans considered the practice of medicine beneath their dignity. Their good fortune was further enhanced when Julius Caesar conferred the full rights of Roman citizenship on all foreign physicians – not that this did anything to improve the quality of their work. Although occasionally a foreigner would rise to a fashionable eminence, most Roman citizens, wisely perhaps, were content to rely on their household gods; when they fell sick they merely consulted the appropriate god and treated themselves with a herbal remedy.

I had no particular urge to visit the Eternal City but Telesphorus was insistent. Late on a summer's morning, walking beside a paved Roman road, we came to a crossroads high in a treeless landscape.

"Let us see where these roads lead," I said, "and then set our faces towards the furthermost." It was as good a way as any of postponing the inevitable.

I sent Telesphorus to consult the milestones. "Rome lies straight ahead... Rome lies to our right... and to our left... we have even come from Rome!" I looked accusingly at him.

"Telesphorus, is this a game you are playing?" I demanded.

"No Master." He was indignant. I walked to the stones myself. True enough, all gave the distance to Rome – and it was the same distance on each stone – yet from where we stood on high ground, I could see the four roads stretching away straight to the horizons in the north, east, south and west.

"Well, my friend, it seems I have no choice. All roads lead to Rome, so to Rome I must go."

I picked up a handful of dust and threw it in the air. It drifted to the west and that was the road we chose.

And now, whether I wished it or no, here we were, Telesphorus and I, bound inevitably for Rome.

*   *   *

I waited at Tivoli while Telesphorus went on to the city to prepare for my arrival. Rome was no place for a newcomer – particularly a physician – lacking an outward display of wealth. But I knew I could rely on Telesphorus to ensure I made a sufficiently dramatic entry.

He returned to announce the acquisition of an imposing residence on the Palatine hill and the seeding of a formidable reputation.

"Galen is most anxious to make your acquaintance." This surprised me as the man was well known to hold his fellow physicians in low regard. "It is more than ten years since he left Alexandria and he wishes to discuss the teaching of his work in the university." That more than explained his interest.

Telesphorus paused; he evidently had not finished his report but I gave him no encouragement to continue; his uncertainty amused me.

"I replied," he hesitated again. "I replied that the greatest physician in Egypt, Paulus Alexandrinus, would be pleased to meet the greatest physician in Rome." The words came in a rush; I had never seen Telesphorus so embarrassed.

"Telesphorus, what else did you say? I know the reputation of this man. His standing as the most – indeed the only – fashionable healer in Rome is such that he believes no other can even aspire to be his equal. And he has wealth, both from his own labours and by inheritance."

"Ah, Master, you see he holds Hippocrates in high esteem and his ambition is to build upon the work of his predecessor, which he says was left unfinished...."

"Yes, yes! I know," I interrupted. "But what did you say that will annoy me?" I was finding Telesphorus's reluctance to come to the point somewhat exasperating.

"...so that he himself will be recognized as the greatest physician the world has known." Telesphorus was not to be hurried. "But he also intends that when he has completed the work begun by Hippocrates, nothing will remain to be discovered and the name of Galen will reign supreme and for ever unchallengable!"

"And what did you say?"

"I told him my master had studied all the books on medicine in the

Alexandrian library and had compiled a summary of all medical knowledge to which he had added his own commentary." Telesphorus's eyes remained firmly fixed on the floor as he related the conversation. "I said this outshone the *De re medicina* since you were a physician and Celsus was not. I also told him you had discovered an unknown text by Hippocrates which you had included in your book and had been able to prove its value in the treatment of your patients."

"Telesphorus! You know I did no such thing!" I was astounded and could only hope that he had some equally facile explanation to extract me from what could be a most difficult situation. "And what text am I supposed to have found?"

"It was only a short one, Master, and concerned with the humours." Telesphorus was almost contrite. "I said you had found a hitherto overlooked passage in *On airs, waters and places* which clarified Hippocrates's views on how changes in the weather affected the balance of the humours in the body and in that way led to disease. It also made it plain that the movements of the heavenly bodies did not, of themselves, cause disease. This, Master, will gratify Galen as it confirms him in his contempt for astrological predictions and magical remedies."

The reputation of Paulus Alexandrinus (I rather liked the authoritative ring of my new name) was secure. If Galen should challenge me, I knew I could match him in any argument about Hippocrates. I also knew that Telesphorus was aware of this and I strongly suspected that it was he who had been amusing himself at *my* expense. He was certainly amused and delighted by the look on my face when he showed me how I was to cover the last few miles into Rome. Outside in the stable yard was a magnificent grey stallion. Its coat was pure unblemished white, immaculately groomed. The cloth across its back was quite plain and secured by a girth. The only ornamentation Telesphorus had deemed fitting for such an animal was confined to the four medallions on the bridle: they were of gold encrusted with precious stones dancing in the early morning sun. The reins of fine leather seemed superfluous, as instinct told me the horse would respond to my slightest movement. I walked up to him and stroked his neck.

"I can almost believe the spirit of Alexander's Bucephalus lives again in this animal," I remarked. Telesphorus grinned and, as if to prove the point, the horse knelt for me to mount. For himself, Telesphorus had purchased a chestnut pony, smaller but no less magnificent in its own form. At length we were on our way, but a final surprise awaited. As we left the complex that was Tivoli, a group of African horsemen cantered up and halted in a clatter of hooves. Their captain saluted then wheeled his troop to ride before us, making our route into the city both clear and safe.

*　　*　　*

Rome was a city with two natures: each in its own way the creation of the other. Despite the congested clamour of its streets, its physical manifestation cast a spell on me from the moment I rode through the Nomentanum gate. Ovid's epithet could not be bettered. The eternal quality he had sensed entered my spirit. But, alas! their own creation was in the process of destroying the creators. It was no longer the Romans who ruled, but the city itself.

As I soon discovered, the population had become exhausted by the perpetual demands of its home; the emperors governed in the name of Rome and through the fear of Rome. The inhabitants of the slums – mostly, and inappropriately, on the dominating Esquiline hill – often found escape from the misery of existence in the collapse of their tenements. The wealthy submitted to the will of Rome, all initiative and inventive vigour drained from them by the requirements of office of one sort or another.

Besides his ability to dissolve time, Telesphorus seemed to have another, less desirable, talent. He had, once again, introduced me to a city ravaged by plague. [This plague is believed to have been smallpox, Dr Annandale. My recollection of its manifestations is poor so I hesitate to offer an opinion; I suspect, though, that like the Thucydidean plague of Athens it also was a compound epidemic. Nevertheless, it is likely that the Roman army, which was severely depleted by the disease, was instrumental in its spread into the distant parts of the Empire. If this was the case, it increases the likelihood that the plague was smallpox rather than a disease of dirt and overcrowding since, if nothing else, the Romans laid great stress on the hygienic well-being of their armies. Any medical benefits thus gained were purely fortuitous!]

When I drew Telesphorus's attention to his unfortunate habit, he merely shrugged his shoulders as if to imply that wherever he took me epidemic disease would not be far away.

"Paulus Alexandrinus," I think he, too, liked the resonance of the name he had given me, "it is time to visit the Illustrious Galen – as some describe him – for he intends to leave the city and I believe you might profit from his commendation."

Galen received me with a degree of circumspection; not every day did he meet a fellow physician with a reputation as impressive as the one Telesphorus had laid on me. At first, as we talked of matters of no consequence, I felt no warmth towards him and could well appreciate how his prodigious intellect would ruffle the feathers of lesser mortals. But when I explained that even though my own knowledge of medicine was unequalled in Alexandria, I had come to Rome to learn the manner in which he had extended the teachings of Hippocrates, his reserve began to fall away.

I sat back and studied him. As we talked on, my first impressions required adjustment as now the true Galen was beginning to appear. He was a driven being; a man fearful in the knowledge that time was not on his side if he was to achieve the divine purpose; for the task he believed the gods had set him was to display the entire fabric of medicine and, through his writings, to lead the world to an understanding of disease. Did he, I wondered, have an over-inflated idea of his own abilities? Or had he been blessed (or, more likely, cursed) with a sufficient intensity of purpose to reach his goal? It did, though, seem to me that if ever a man possessed the necessary mental equipment, it was Galen. Yet beneath his intellectual and practical skills lay an indefinable quality that served to explain his popularity among those fortunate to experience this aspect of his character. I saw now why Telesphorus had been so anxious that I should meet him – and on terms as near equal as Galen would allow.

Then I noticed that he, in turn, had been studying me. His face held much the same expression as had been in Themison's quizzical gaze. And, like Themison, Galen, too, was unable to find what he was seeking, though he saw enough to take me into his confidence.

"I have always been suspicious," he said, "of those who maintain that disease is sent by the gods through the movements of the planets. My own belief," and his voice made it plain that it was more than belief, "is that disease is caused by an imbalance of the humours brought about by changes in the diet or in the weather or by differences in the climate from one region to another. But, Paulus, your... your...." Telesphorus's status had evidently bewildered him.

"Telesphorus is my student and assistant," I helped him out.

"Yes. Your assistant tells me you have discovered an unknown work of Hippocrates." He smiled for the first time. It came slowly, as if rarely permitted. Indeed, I suspected that it was only permitted when there was something to be gained. At this point I was in half a mind to keep my "discovery" to myself, but the other half decided to accept Telesphorus's judgment that Galen was a man worth cultivating. I withdrew from my sleeve a document I had written in the Hippocratic style the previous evening.

"I made a copy of a passage not known to scholars – certainly I can find no mention of it in the works of Celsus." So saying I handed him the sheet of vellum I had used for my deception. He read it. He read it again.

"Paulus!" He gripped my hand – he was not given to shows of emotion. "This gives the lie to those who argue against me. We are truly, every one of us, individuals who must be treated as such when ill." [You will see, Dr Annandale, how strict adherence to the doctrine of the humours denied the possibility of disease being spread by contagion – the sole responsible factor was held to be individual susceptibility to humoral change. Yet many veterinarians were well aware of contagion among animals and Virgil wrote of the spread of anthrax in sheep from herd to herd. Nothing could prick the intellectual arrogance of the medical fraternity; anything that did not fit with their theories was discarded.]

"Now I can go further. But first, you can assure me that this is a true copy of what you read and that the writer was indeed Hippocrates?"

I think I could have said that the writer was the great god Pluto and he would still have accepted it, such was his desire to be proved correct. Nevertheless, I gave a true answer: "It was beyond any doubt written by one of the Hippocratic school of physicians."

"Then I am indebted to you. I have been labouring to show that the balance of a man's humours is reflected in his temperament. And this passage indicates clearly that Hippocrates was of like mind, although he does not commit himself to a plain statement."

With difficulty I hid my perplexity. I had not the least idea of his meaning. I need not have worried.

"A man's temperament," he continued without pause, "is soon discovered by the watchful physician. The treatment of sickness is to restore the equilibrium of the humours."

He then launched headlong into an account of his correlation of the humours with human characteristics.

The truth of what I say walks the streets of Rome as, indeed, they do of any city," he began. "Those who are of a fiery, swift and passionate nature and are given to silent rages have the sanguine temperament; their constitution is hot and humid and they are ruled by the blood of their humours. Many native inhabitants of this country are of a sanguine temperament. When they fall sick they are to be treated with medicines possessed of a similar temperament. Dill and fenugreek are of the first order since their heat is imperceptible to the senses. Caustics are of the fourth and last order."

Scarcely pausing for breath, he pounded his way through the other three temperaments, the choleric, the melancholic and the phlegmatic. "Those of a choleric disposition are given to anger and pride; they have a hot and dry constitution and their ruling humour is yellow bile. You yourself will have noticed that many Egyptians are of this temperament. The melancholic and phlegmatic, being of a cold nature, are found most often in the tribes along the northern frontiers of the Empire. The melancholic are cold and dry and the phlegmatic cold and humid. In the first order of cooling medicines is rose oil and the rose itself; in the second is the juice of roses; in the third and fourth are those medicines that are extremely cold and amongst which I number meconium, mandragora and hyoscyamus. It is necessary to chose and combine our medicines in such a manner as shall render them effective in overcoming the varied conditions that exist in different diseases."

Suddenly he changed his tone. "Come with me," he commanded – I was left with no choice.

He led me through his house to a large room opening onto a colonnaded garden, resplendent with a rich variety of flowers, herbs and shrubs. But it was not the garden that drew my attention, it was the contents of the room itself. It was filled with containers of all shapes and sizes and all carefully labelled.

"I use opium, mandragora and hyoscyamus to narcotize severe pain," he said, pointing to each of the containers in turn. "In this I follow the teachings of Hippocrates. But," and here a note of triumph entered his voice, "I have carried forward his understanding of pain. Pain does not come only from outside causes – as when a man is wounded by arrows or swords, or stung by venomous beasts, or burned by fire. No! pain may also arise from the organs within the body and so give warning to the physician that he would be well advised to administer an agreeable remedy. You found no mention of inner pain in the works of Hippocrates or the writings of Celsus?" I admitted that, no, I had not.

Meanwhile, my eyes had been wandering round the shelves. Everything seemed to be in keeping with his Hippocratic protestations until my gaze lighted, first, on a jar labelled "Fox oil" and a moment or two later on another, smaller, container stating "Dried camel brain". Even the Illustrious Galen was not immune to the legacy of folk-lore.

Hiding my scepticism, I asked what use he found for these preparations.

"I obtain the fox oil by boiling foxes and use it as a bath to ease the aching of painful joints – you have no use for it in Alexandria?" He spoke in all seriousness. I shook my head. "And the dried camel brain, I give in vinegar as a welcome cure for epilepsy – the sacred disease of Hippocrates. And there," he pointed at a glass vessel decorated with gold and containing a concoction resembling nothing so much as a long-forgotten meal, "there you see a favourite remedy for diseases afflicting the skin. It is vipers' flesh specially and most carefully prepared. When required, I shall put it up in pastilles." He went on to explain how the viper owed its excellence to the fact that it shed its skin. When boiled in wine or vinegar, he said, the skin itself was a remedy for toothache and earache, though the rationale for this escaped me – as it did Galen!

It must have been the bemused expression on my face at the sheer quantity of medicines arranged in ordered sequence that prompted his next remark.

"Yes," he said, "drugs are sent to me from Palestine, Syria, Egypt, Pontus, Macedonia, Cappadocia, Spain, Gaul, Africa – from all over the world. Every one I examine meticulously to ensure that it is of the correct variety and age. And, again, before I administer a medicine, I study it closely for though twins may look alike to a stranger, they are easily distinguished by those who know them."

Then, to my amazement, he swept his arm around the shelves: "As you can see, I am running short of many drugs and shall soon have to travel for more!" He stopped; evidently an idea had come unexpectedly upon him. He looked hard at me.

"I cannot leave immediately as the Emperor has entrusted his son to my care and no other physician in Rome is worthy of the responsibility. But," and he looked at me again; he could see in me that quality that so perplexed yet reassured him. "I believe Marcus Aurelius would find you acceptable. I have business at home in Pergamum and on the way I mean to obtain minerals from the copper mines in Cyprus – I have no flowers of zinc for treating weeping malignant ulcers. Also, on my return I intend to visit the Dead Sea to collect a fresh supply of asphalt." This did not surprise me as Galen's reputation for the treatment of gladiatorial wounds owed much to his use of this bituminous substance which he applied with a sponge and set alight. As often as not the bleeding took fright and stopped.

[Galen is sometimes accused of having left Rome to escape the plague, but this is unlikely as the epidemic was flourishing in Pergamum as it was all over the Empire. Another story is that he was fleeing from the hatred of his physician rivals. Both these excuses ring false and would have been completely out of character. I see no reason, Dr Annandale, to doubt what he told me although, admittedly, I did not know him well at this time.]

And so it was that a few days later Galen summoned me (there is no other word for it) to attend the Emperor Marcus Aurelius with him. It was a meeting that proved to be the start of a profound change in my life. Not in its course; that alas! was something I was powerless to alter; I had to flow wherever the tide of medicine chose to sweep me. No, it was my attitude to life – or more particularly, if I am to be honest, to women – that underwent a none-too-subtle alteration. I suppose at that time I must have appeared as a man of twenty-five or thirty years. My relationships with women had been very much that of passing ships bound for diverse ports and even when I believed I had caught a fleeting glimpse of my Ishtar, the horizon soon engulfed her to leave me alone again in the silent darkness. For my part the emotional turmoil of our closeness was sorely lacking in maturity.

*   *   *

The walk from my home to the Tiberian House was short. How Telesphorus had acquired a villa so conveniently close to the imperial residence would remain his secret, though of one thing I could be sure: the transaction would have been perfectly honourable. The morning was already hot, even for late August – the date is fixed in my mind since Lucius Verus, co-emperor with Marcus, had earlier that month returned victorious from the east. It was one of life's ironies that he, the supreme commander, had been gaming and sporting in Syria, while Statius Priscus had been fighting the battles in Armenia and Avidius Cassius those beyond the Tigris. But Lucius's winnings at dice had not been all he had picked up in Syria: he had acquired a mistress of outstanding beauty and superior intelligence. Her name was Panthea. Such was her influence over him that she even persuaded him to shave off the beard of which he was inordinately proud!

Marcus received me with a natural charm, almost as if we were old friends meeting again after a long absence, though beneath the warmth there lay the austere seriousness of the Stoic philosopher. Despite having long abandoned the athletic pursuits of his youth, he still retained a litheness of body and an ease of movement. In some inexplicable manner he reminded me of the young Alexander before the lust of conquest became rooted in his soul. It was Marcus's attitude to me that drew the comparison – certainly it was not a physical resemblance since his curly dark-brown hair grew long over his forehead and ears and merged into an equally curly beard and a neatly trimmed moustache. His wide-apart deep-set eyes held a look that told of an inner orderliness and determination.

I waited for the Emperor to speak while he studied me closely but with no hint of discourtesy.

"You *are* Paulus Alexandrinus?" he enquired at length.

"Yes," I assured him.

"Your reputation has preceded you. If I am to release my physician," he glanced at Galen who had been standing at his side since my arrival, "from his imperial duties, I must needs replace him with another of comparable worth – and he speaks well of you. Apollonius taught me to recognize a man who would treat life seriously and yet remain comfortably at ease. I recognize such a man in you. He also taught me to be immutable at the loss of a child. That was a hard lesson, for I have lost six children, five of them sons. I do not wish that Commodus and Annius should follow their brothers."

We were about to leave when Marcus stopped me and with a look that I can only describe as quizzically humorous, asked for my opinion on the plague.

"There are some," I answered after a pause in which I struggled to determine the motive underlying the question, "who hold Cassius responsible on account of his sacking of Seleucia after the city had welcomed the Roman army as friends. But that I do not believe as treaties have been violated before without such terrible consequences. Nor do I believe the Christians have brought the pestilence upon us. I agree with the people that it has been sent by the gods – and I do not choose to seek an explanation for their actions."

"Then we are all in agreement!" So saying, he motioned that we might withdraw.

Annius, the younger of the two boys by a year, was of a gentle disposition and treated almost as a doll by his four elder sisters. The five-year-old Commodus was another matter; I took an immediate aversion to him which was intensified when I experienced his tantrums and outbursts of vicious temper. These, in my more charitable moments, I attributed to the death of his twin brother some months previously. I did not, however, take a similar aversion to his mother.

Faustina was the most beautiful woman I had encountered for many a long year. Yet there was more to her beauty than the pure physical perfection so admired by the Greeks; there was an unsettling sensuality about her, which tragedy had served only to heighten, that tore at my loins. It explained why men desired to possess her and why, I suspect, she would have spent her life in one long and glorious pregnancy.

After our first meeting, my loins were in tatters and the voice of experience informed me that, had the children not been present, she would have welcomed an attempt on my part to have saved them from their temporary ruin. Although we met again many times, on no other occasion was I moved to such an extreme; I will not deny the existence of a certain physical excitement in her presence, but she could not reach my heart. She was not to be a second Roxana. Nevertheless, I found my emotional relationship with her to be a disturbing experience as she was the first woman whose sensuality had the power to scare me. I can think of no other way to express the effect she had on me at that time. But as she was Augusta and the mother of Commodus and Annius, I could not escape. I resolved to serve her for the sake of Marcus Aurelius and for no other reason.

In the middle of October, the two Emperors were awarded a triumph – the first for fifty years – for the victories in the east. But if the eastern frontiers of the Empire were secure, trouble was brewing in the north beyond the Danube. At the turn of the year, two of the tribes invaded Pannonia, not for their customary pleasure in raping and pillaging, but to gain much-needed land. Despite their being rapidly beaten back, Marcus announced that he would go north to discover the situation for himself. This, I was sure, was ill-advised considering the mood of the Roman people. During the winter months the plague had increased in virulence and was carrying off many thousands of citizens, making no distinction between wretched plebeian and noble patrician – except that the most eminent among the latter had statues erected to their memory. The Emperor's presence was urgently required in Rome to maintain the morale of his people.

When the rumour began to spread that the plague was divine retribution – though for what, was never made clear – rather than a mere whim of the gods, the citizens demanded that something should be done, I saw my opportunity and suggested a number of laws and proscriptions on the transport of bodies and the burial of the dead, all of which the Emperors enacted. [I doubt, Dr Annandale, whether Galen would even have thought of these measures as they implied an acceptance of contagion. However, Marcus accepted them on my assurances that Virgil and other writers had found similar precautions of value.]

Yet the plague continued to wreak destruction and in view of what I had originally said to Marcus, I considered it only right to suggest that he should summon the priests to purify the city. He agreed with enthusiasm which led me to suspect that he had already made the decision. The traditional rites concluded with the celebration by the Emperors of the ancient ceremony of the feast of the gods – this required that statues of the gods be lain on banqueting couches in the city's public places with offerings placed on tables beside them. The celebration continued for seven days with benefit only to the gods. At this Marcus, unintentionally I think, showed me the nature of his concern for humanity.

"Paulus," he said while we were deliberating what further steps he could take, "corruption of the mind is a far greater pestilence than any corruption and change of the air that surrounds us." (This view that disease might originate from a corruption of the air echoed the teachings of Hippocrates which Marcus had doubtless learnt from Galen.) "For this corruption," he continued, referring to the plague, "is a pestilence of men in so far as they are animals; corruption of the mind is a pestilence of men in so far as they are human beings."

That evening as I sat in silent companionship with Telesphorus, I wondered whether the mind was, indeed, of greater importance than the body. I was uncertain whether the Emperor had been speaking literally of human morality or whether he had been inferring that in his philosophy physical disease had its origins in a corruption of the mind. If this were so, and he was right, the search for an understanding of disease must begin with the mind.

"And there's the problem of the Christians." Telesphorus broke in on my reverie. "In the past, they have been persecuted for their beliefs and for their refusal to honour and propitiate the ancient gods of Rome. Now they are the perfect scapegoat. Why could they not have joined in the ceremonies simply out of respect for the Emperors? But no! they have chosen to make themselves conspicuous by their blatant disbelief. 'Those unwilling to sacrifice to the gods, after being scourged, are to be executed in accordance with the laws'," he quoted. "The people say that it is downright obstinacy on their part; that they want to become martyrs."

"Marcus wouldn't agree with that," I said, trying to recall his exact words to me. "He thinks it is something that goes beyond a willingness to die. Ah! I have it now: 'How wonderful is a soul that, at the very moment when it is to be released from the body, is prepared to be no more, to be scattered in pieces, or to survive in some other form. But,' and he was emphatic here, 'this preparedness must come from a specific decision and not from sheer parataxis* like the Christians. They choose to die,' he said, 'not through free-will but because they have been trained to be ready for death.' "

* Parataxis is a Greek word that in those days referred, inter alia, to the drawing-up of troops in battle. Although a suitable meaning in this context could be "obstinacy", the military allusion of parataxis makes Marcus's choice particularly apt. – J.G.

7

...The man who would discover and record all medical knowledge*

Before the year was out, Galen returned to Rome and, whether he wished it or not, I continued to serve the Imperial family. I had certainly gained the confidence of Marcus with my sound medical knowledge and regard for his Stoic philosophy. Although Faustina still disturbed my loins, we understood each other. Despite her indiscretions – which were few, contrary to popular rumour – she was devoted to her husband and was aware of my loyalty to him.

Galen, strangely for a man so self-centred and so condemnatory of his fellows, welcomed my assistance, particularly at his anatomy demonstrations. Even so, he could go just so far and no further – he gave me no credit, either in writing or through the spoken word, for a number of accurate observations I made. But at least I was not expected to skin his monkeys for him – he now did this himself after one of his slaves had removed some underlying muscle at the same time. These demonstrations attracted many curious patricians, including Marcus himself.

As far as Galen was concerned, Aristotle's belief that Nature made nothing in vain was the ultimate truth. So, as every anatomical structure must have been designed for a definite purpose, Galen reasoned that if he could identify these structures their purpose would immediately be clear. The first – and only – time I challenged one of his conclusions

*Galen continues as physician to Marcus Aurelius. 169-177. – J.G.

he told me, in a voice like the wind off a frozen peak:

"The human body is the work of the Creator. He has made even the most inaccessible of its parts to work in harmony, one with another. Each action of the body has its cause. When a cause is out of harmony, there is discord and function is lost – the body is injured or becomes diseased."

That was that. Galen had spoken and there was to be no argument. [Do not be misled, Dr Annandale, by Galen's reference to a Creator. This had no religious significance – he was talking about Aristotle's Nature.] His technical skill at dissection was impressive and, as he proceeded, seven scribes recorded his descriptions not only of what he found – which was usually accurate – but also his perception of its function – which was frequently speculative, if not downright fanciful. Speaking anatomically, his greatest deficiency lay with the subjects of his dissections. Only rarely did a human corpse come his way – and even then its value was, as like as not, reduced to the study of its skeleton. But this was of small concern to him. What the Creator had created in the beast, that had He also created in man. So Galen, with supreme indifference, dissected apes (whose right kidneys lie higher than their left), dogs (the disposition of whose livers makes them appear to have five lobes), pigs, sheep and other animals besides, all of whose individual anatomical quirks were solemnly recorded as being human attributes.

On the occasion when I challenged him, he was demonstrating the heart and blood vessels in a goat and expounding on their purpose and that of the blood.

"Blood is created in the liver. Here also the vena cava has its beginning, that it may transport the blood to the right side of the heart. From this side it passes through pores – which I cannot demonstrate as they are too small to be visible to the human eye – into the left ventricle where it becomes charged with pneuma." Galen looked up and paused to assure himself that he had the attention of his audience.

"Why do we breathe?" The question was shot out in a seeming change of direction. No one was inclined to answer. "Because the air enters the lungs where it is partly changed into vital pneuma," he continued. "From the lungs it travels through the pulmonary veins to the left ventricle where the process of conversion to vital pneuma is completed by the heat of the heart. The blood is now redder and thinner than when it was created in the liver. But this change produces sooty vapours which travel back along the pulmonary veins to the lungs and are expelled in the breath."

Galen pointed to the valve [the mitral valve, Dr Annandale] at the entrance to the left ventricle before proceeding. "The purpose of this structure," he explained, "is to permit the sooty vapours to pass into the pulmonary veins while preventing the blood from doing likewise.

"The blood in the left ventricle is now fully charged with vital pneuma and is propelled by the heart to all parts of the body where it is entirely consumed." Galen moved to the animal's head where I had been busy dissecting the base of its brain. I had displayed the rete mirabile, a network of blood vessels and nerves peculiar to ungulates.

"The rete mirabile has a great purpose." Galen pronounced the statement with all the weight of a line from a Homeric epic. "In the rete mirabile, the vital pneuma is transmuted into psychic pneuma! This flows into the brain and into the nerves. It is psychic pneuma that gives sensation and imparts movement!" It was all so simple and logical and clearly explained to the Galenic mind why the structures we had dissected had been created.

*   *   *

In the spring, Marcus and Lucius, clad in the military cloak, left Rome for Aquileia* where they arrived to find the frontier tribes either pacified or defeated. Instead the threat to Rome came yet again from the plague. The army had suffered badly – indeed, there were those who said it had been destroyed, almost to the point of annihilation.

When Galen received the summons to join the Imperial staff, I decided to keep him company. Although his labours to control the plague were in vain, the presence of the Emperors and the two greatest physicians in the Roman Empire had a steadying effect on the army.

"There is little now to be gained by both of us remaining here," Lucius made the suggestion to Marcus as spring gave way to summer. "Rome has need of your talents and I can exercise command alone." This, he knew, would make few demands on his time; his intention, once he had seen Marcus on the road to Rome was to leave administrative matters to his staff while he indulged in a flurry of hunting and feasting with Panthea to soothe his tired body. He was

* Later the site of Venice. – J.G.

not one to allow the plague – or the demands of office – to interfere with his pleasures.

But it was not to be. Marcus was firm in his determination to secure the northern frontier. Since he saw the present cessation of hostilities as a barbarian ruse to put the Romans off their guard, he manoeuvred an unwilling Lucius across the Alps to Carnuntum*. From here, he meticulously laid plans for carrying the offensive into tribal territories the following spring.

While we were at Carnuntum, there were the inevitable minor skirmishes which I mention only because they gave me the opportunity to observe Galen, the wound surgeon. His ability was beyond reproach – as I suppose was to be expected of a man who claimed never to have lost a wounded gladiator while working in his younger days at the arena of his native Pergamum. [Believe this if you will, Dr Annandale! I imagine he selected only those who showed no inclination to die. There is a parallel here, too, with certain practices on offer in your world.] One aspect of his treatment intrigued me: he regarded suppuration – or coction, as he called it – to be part of the natural healing of wounds. He never made it clear, certainly not to me, whether this was a consequence of a belief in the doctrine of the humours, with the wounded body ridding itself of excess phlegm, or whether it was the fruit of experience. A clue that it might have been the latter came when he asked:

"Have you, Paulus, noticed how the soldier whose wound does not undergo coction and who develops a raging fever usually dies, whereas the one whose wound does undergo coction is more likely to live?"

I had to admit that, no, I had not – which was the truth.

[Once again, Dr Annandale, Galen was drawing a logical conclusion from the facts available to him. He had noticed two different types of wound infection – which you would recognize as caused by different types of bacteria. He looked upon suppuration as a good thing since it meant that probably the more lethal wound infection was not going to occur and, though he could not realize this, the suppuration was helping to get rid of any dirt, dead tissue or foreign body, that might have been driven into the wound.]

Recrossing the Alps, the Emperors prepared to winter at Aquileia,

---

* On the Danube about twenty miles east of the modern Vienna. – J.G.

but it was cold and wet and the plague still held the town in a fearsome grip. Galen advised a return to Rome, particularly as Marcus was not in the best of health, and at the start of the year the Imperial suite set out. Yet it was not Marcus whom Atropos chose for her victim.

We had travelled for no more than two days and had reached Altinum when Lucius was struck with an apoplexy. Three days later he was dead. Marcus continued the journey with the body.

Once the funeral ceremonies and all the religious obligations due the dead Emperor and his family had been disposed of, Marcus moved events forward with all speed. He was acutely aware of the importance of extending the Roman conquests beyond the Danube to discourage barbarian aggression. He restored the army to fighting strength by recruiting new legions from an assortment of slaves, bandits, provincial mercenaries and (to the annoyance of the people of Rome) gladiators. To finance the undertaking he was compelled to hold a two-month auction of Imperial chattels and personal jewellery and to devalue the currency – the imposition of further taxation would have been perilously unpopular.

With matters military well in hand, Marcus had still to deal with the immediate family problems created by Lucius's death: in brief, what to do about Lucilla, his own daughter and Lucius's widow. Marcus intended that he himself should be succeeded by Commodus (this would be the first time in Imperial history that a son had succeeded his father – and, in my opinion it was one of the rare occasions when Marcus was guilty of a serious error of judgment by allowing the love for that son to outweigh his duty to his country), but whoever married Lucilla, the minor Augusta, would be in an extremely strong position to displace the disastrous Commodus. A number of names, among them the Syrian, Avidius Cassius, suggested themselves only to be discarded as too much of a threat – particularly that of Cassius whose family could claim descent from eastern royalty. In the end, Marcus settled for a safe alternative: Claudius Pompeianus, an experienced soldier and former governor of a northern province; his merit lay in his being of only minor noble stock. Unfortunately Faustina disliked him to the point of loathing and the mourning nineteen-year-old who was to be the recipient of her father's politicking confided in me that she would almost rather take her own life – Pompeianus was over fifty! No amount of pleading by either woman would shake Marcus's determination and, long before the required period of mourning was ended, the young widow was married.

But the gods exacted vengeance. While Marcus was imposing his will on the rest of his family, Annius was operated on (not, need I say it, by either Galen or myself) for a "tumour" behind his ear and died soon after. [I suspect, Dr Annandale, that the "tumour" was the inflammatory swelling of mastoiditis. I have often since wondered how the course of history might have changed had Annius lived to pose a challenge to Commodus who was to become a greater curse to Rome than any pestilence or crime.] In both public and private, Marcus behaved with true Stoic self-control and gave no outward sign of the depth of his grief.

He still had one more responsibility to attend to before returning north: the neutralization of any threat that Panthea might pose. Though he knew her well enough to believe her incapable of treason, danger would lurk in the shape of the man she chose to marry. She had grieved bitterly, more from the loss of status the relationship had brought her than from love of Lucius, and she was now in obvious need of consolation.

I was attending the Emperor at the Circus games in September when, discussing mourning in general and Panthea's and his own mother's in particular, he remarked:

"And if they were still sitting by the tomb, would the dead notice? And if they did notice, would they be pleased? And if they were pleased, would that make them immortal? Paulus, you are a handsome man and an intellectual match for Panthea. You would help her to forget Lucius and," he smiled knowingly, "she would be a great comfort to you – I have seen the looks that passed between you when Lucius was away."

So Panthea and I were married with the Imperial blessing and, as it proved, to the great comfort of us both. Since, if I were to describe her qualities myself, I would be accused of exaggeration, I must paint her portrait in the words of Lucian, a man not given to unwonted flattery: She was a woman of perfect beauty, more beautiful even than any statue by Phidias or Praxiteles. Her voice was soft, delicious and winning; she spoke pure Ionic Greek with the savour of Attic wit; she sang wondrously to the lyre. She was possessed of the gifts of all the Muses; she had a shrewd understanding of public affairs. She was gracious, loving and modest by nature.

(Oh! my Ishtar, are you but an illusion, a mere fantasy that I can forget you in the arms of another?)

Marcus had had us married with the same indecent haste as he had had Lucilla. Nevertheless, it was October before all the domestic and administrative details were in place and the Imperial party was ready to leave. The campaigning season may have been over, but Marcus had in mind the launching of a mighty offensive to initiate the next.

Amongst those he took with him were Pompeianus, newly appointed his chief military adviser, and Lucilla, Panthea and myself. Galen was also ordered to join his staff, but he was loathe to leave his lucrative Roman practice.

"I was able to persuade him, good natured and charitable as he is, to leave me at Rome," he said and I did not need an astrologer to tell me what he would say next. "He was pleased to have you in my stead. I shall meantime continue to supervise the care of Commodus. Now that the boy is his only son, the Emperor would entrust him to no one but myself should he fall ill!"

I chose to ignore the contradiction in what he said and the implied contempt of myself. There was no arguing with the man when he was in one of his boastful moods. In any case, before I could think of a suitable retort, he was lecturing me on the peculiarities of the Emperor's own health – most of which I had discovered on our previous expedition.

"You need not worry overmuch as, indeed, he will soon return," he concluded. If anyone needed the help of an astrologer it was Galen; only if he regarded seven years as soon, would his prediction come true.

Marcus was, I believe, genuinely fond of Panthea and myself and we enjoyed many a discussion and argument. But the longer I spent in his company, the more concerned I became about his health. His physical weakness was even more in evidence than the previous winter and he would often order a review of the legions and scarcely have left his quarters before retiring again. The damp coldness was something he found hard to endure.

"Why," I asked, "will you not return to Rome as last year? Pompeianus is trustworthy and will see your orders are obeyed."

"There is a saying of Epicurus," he replied in his customary oblique fashion, "that should help you understand why I choose not to take your advice. He said that pain was neither unbearable nor unending, so long as we remembered its limitations and did not increase it with our imagination. To this I would add only that what we cannot bear takes us away from life; what lasts can be borne! This war is a harsh necessity for the Roman state. It possesses none of the glory of past conquests. You yourself have seen the confidence of our soldiers eroded by the pestilence. I have to remain with them."

Marcus ate only at night and would take nothing during the day except the theriac which, at his request, Galen had compounded for him. Galen's theriac was like none other! He doubled the number of ingredients to one hundred, and instructed that it be taken in honey and wine. It was, he maintained, a remarkable remedy for all internal afflictions, especially those of the stomach. It certainly eased the pains in Marcus's chest and stomach but at the expense of making him drowsy – due, no doubt, to the quantity of opium it contained! Galen was nobody's fool. When he stopped taking the remedy, Marcus was unable to sleep and his pains returned. So it was back to the theriac. This told me how intense the pains must have been, yet Marcus, a Stoic of no mean fortitude, made no complaint.

*   *   *

I stayed in the north as one of the Imperial suite for two years. Despite the horror of Roman soldiers killing, raping, pillaging and burning, seemingly in a spirit of senseless revenge at the never-ending destruction of their own lives by the plague, Panthea and I delighted in each other, both physically and intellectually. I found her to be the kindest, most understanding, most desirable of women. So marked was the contrast between her gentle sensuality and the raw sexuality of Faustina that when the Empress arrived at headquarters, I took flight back to Rome. This met with Panthea's enthusiastic approval; her Syrian constitution did not relish the prospect of another Danube winter.

We found Galen immersed in one of his frequent and furious bouts of writing. His commitment to the recording of all medical knowledge verged on the obscene: he shamelessly took as his own whatever extracts from the writings of his predecessors suited his purpose and without any attribution to their source. But he argued that his own discoveries, particularly in regard to the physiology of the nervous system, carried knowledge so far forward that any reference to the past was superfluous – and would, indeed, confuse matters.

At the time of our return, he was engaged in describing his pulse lore which he considered to be a cornerstone of the practice of medicine. In all, this required the writing of sixteen books, divided into four groups: the differences between pulses; the causes of pulsation; the diagnoses revealed by the pulses; and the prognoses to be derived from the pulses. [Even he, Dr Annandale, eventually appreciated that this was too much to stomach, and twenty years later he produced a single-volume summary. He insisted on explaining to me the reasoning behind the lore in considerable detail, but rather than use his own words I have chosen to give a short résumé. You will probably find it rather incomprehensible, though to Galen it was, as always, totally logical.]

According to Galen, both the heart and the arteries beat individually but simultaneously. Expansion and contraction of the arteries were distinct active, as opposed to passive, movements. Expansion drew in pneuma derived from the inspiration of atmospheric air (echoes of Erasistratus!) which then became mixed with blood in the heart to become vital pneuma. Contraction helped to expel the sooty vapours. (It was as if the arteries and the lungs worked together toward the same ends.) Consequently, said Galen, the condition of the artery – whether it was hard or soft, for instance – was most important since the pulse was created in the arterial wall and was dependent on vital pneuma.

"The pulse, the arteries, the heart and disease," he had come to the end of his dissertation, "are inextricably linked. Grasp the existence of this relationship and understand the significance of the different manifestations of the pulse and you will be a good physician." (Even if it entailed having to read his sixteen books!) I refrained from telling him – he probably knew, anyway – that Praxagoras about five hundred years before had been aware of the relationship and that it had later been a feature of Alexandrian medicine.

Galen was able to give me a practical demonstration of the value of his pulse lore sooner than either of us expected. He had just finished talking when a messenger arrived from Pitholaus, Commodus's tutor, to say the boy was ill.

"He has come back from a wrestling class with a sore throat and fever," said the tutor in response to Galen's questioning. "I gave him a gargle."

Galen laid his fingers on the boy's wrist. "Commodus has an inflammation. Where is the gargle?"

Pitholaus gave Galen a look of surprised admiration. "I didn't know that inflammation of the tonsils could alter the pulse," he said under his breath, pointing to a flask.

Galen dipped his finger into the solution and tasted it. "Too strong," he said. "Give him instead honey and rosewater."

And on the morning of the third day, the fever had abated.

With the sixteenth book of his pulse lore completed, Galen continued to write or to dictate to his scribes. I had entered his room during a pause for refreshment when he suddenly looked at me and asked in a tone almost of despair:

"What do you make of these followers of Moses and Christ? They live through faith rather than reason. The Christians draw their faith from parables and miracles, and yet some act in the manner of philosophers. Their contempt for death is obvious every day."

As I failed to see where his questioning was leading, I gave a non-committal answer. "They believe that if they are scourged and beheaded, they will rise up into heaven," I said. "No; it is more than a belief, it is a conviction. If they are punished, they *will* be saved. They go to their execution glorifying their God in the name of their Saviour, even though they know that if they repent, they will be pardoned. I don't understand them."

"And *you* don't understand *me*!" Galen was piqued at what he saw as my obtuseness. "If the beliefs of the Christians take hold, they will undermine the science that is at the foundation of medicine. They believe in miracles, but there can be no such thing in an ordered and stable universe. Our patients are healed through knowledge and understanding, not through miracles! Their recovery is proof, not only of our medical skill but also of the Creator's purpose which allows us to proceed logically in an organized world. If this were not so, chaos would reign and all my work would be in vain!"

What had begun as a mild discourse ended with Galen, passionately angry, pacing up and down banging fist into open palm to emphasize each point of his argument. His scribes had already left when they saw how the situation was developing and at one turn when his back was towards me I, too, slipped from the room.

By good fortune – or so it seemed when the Imperial letter arrived – I did not have to face Galen again for some months. The Empress summoned me to Sirmium out of concern for Marcus's health; she preferred my opinion to Galen's. With no reason to suspect the command to be other than it seemed, I set out the following week, misery in my heart at leaving Panthea.

Marcus was in reasonable spirits when I arrived, and I chided Faustina for having brought me on a wasted journey. Reassured, I prepared to return. Faustina, however, took the first opportunity of Marcus's absence from the camp to speak to me alone.

"We are different creatures, you and I," she began, "though we both love the Emperor." With that there could be no argument. "He *was* ill during the worst of the winter and I feared he would die. That is why I sent for you. Not," she hurried on, "to give him physic. If he dies, Pompeianus, as husband of the minor Augusta would be sure to become Commodus's and my protector. This prospect does not appeal to me. The fact that I dislike him is not my point. His right is unquestioned, but I do not see him as equal to the task. Our lives would be in danger and the Emperor's wish that Commodus should succeed him would come to nothing. There is only one man I trust to save us. You will carry a message to Avidius Cassius. I trust you, too, and you will arouse no suspicion travelling to Syria, intending to continue to Alexandria."

She took me by the hand; strangely, I experienced no thrill of excitement. Panthea's love had quite stilled any response I might once have had to Faustina's touch. Her look was one of innocent pleading – *that*, I could not resist.

"You will be doing the Emperor a service only his widow and son will be able to acknowledge." She kissed me, knowing I would not refuse.

I duly delivered the letter.

Cassius's response was, to say the least, dramatic and took me completely by surprise: He immediately had himself proclaimed, and was accepted as, Emperor in Syria and most of the other eastern provinces and, by the end of April, in Egypt.

My first thought was that he had misunderstood Faustina's message and believed Marcus already dead. Then a second, more unpleasant possibility came to mind: could Faustina, for reasons best known to herself, have incited Cassius to rebel? I had not read the letter and as speculation in such a situation is fruitless and likely to lead to more harm than good, I made my way back north with all speed. Cassius made no attempt to have me stopped, even though he had been informed that Marcus was alive.

While Syria gave him unreserved support, its northern neighbour, Cappadocia, remained loyal. When I reported to the governor, Martius Verus, and told him what I knew of the rebellion, he prepared a despatch for Marcus and entrusted it to my care.

Marcus was thunderstruck. In one breath, he abandoned personal command and gave precise orders for others to continue the hostilities. In the next, he summoned Commodus from Rome to join him at Sirmium. And with the next, he began his cross-examination of me. Why had I been in Smyrna? What was the content of Faustina's letter? Why had I not consulted him before going? How committed were the eastern legions to Cassius? Was Martius Verus loyal? But most of all he wanted answers to questions that I could not possibly give. Why had Cassius behaved as he had? Why had he continued with the rebellion when he knew Marcus was still alive?

"Why did my dearest friend turn against me? I made him governor of Syria and gave him command in all the eastern provinces. Had it been the will of the army or of the senate, the Empire could have been his. I continue to labour only for the common good though I am already old and weak and unable to take food without pain or to sleep undisturbed.

"If he did wrong, the evil is on his side; but perhaps he did no wrong"

To my great relief, he accepted Faustina's explanation for her writing to Cassius as he had himself truly believed that he had been on the threshold of death. My concern was that the news might break him. But I should have known better.

Without delay he began the necessary preparations to suppress the rebellion, but before he could set out, a despatch arrived reporting the death of Cassius at the hands of a loyal centurion. Martius Verus had assumed control in Syria and (to my even greater relief) had burned all Cassius's letters. (I have often wondered whether he did this because he had read them; if so, he took his secrets to the grave.) Despite this, Marcus continued with his plans as it was vital to re-establish the loyalty of the eastern provinces.

Roman domination across the Danube enabled Marcus to conclude peace with the barbarians and be free to travel east. He took with him Faustina, Commodus and, under protest, myself – I wanted to return to Rome; I had been away from Panthea for the best part of a year.

There was a little village in Cappadocia by the name of Halala nestling in the foothills of the Taurus mountains, the name of which, for the rest of his life was carved deeply into the heart of Marcus Aurelius. It was winter again, and even he had to agree it was no place for a woman. Faustina was forty-five years old and whether she was again pregnant I cannot say, but the journey was more than her body could support. At Halala, she died. Marcus could find no words that would express his grief. He loved her and, in what to him was a thoroughly inadequate memorial, he renamed the village Faustinopolis.

I left Marcus to continue his progress throughout the east while I returned to Rome and Panthea.

Galen's reputation, already remarkable for a Greek physician in the Roman Empire, continued to grow. His success with his patients – although not necessarily with the cure of their diseases – was owed in large measure to his practice of explaining the nature of the illness, including the prognosis, and gaining the patient's understanding of the treatment he prescribed.

I had one last opportunity to see and marvel at his skill before tragedy overtook me. At the end of the year it was a sick Marcus who returned with his son. The physicians who accompanied him had diagnosed a violent fever and prescribed rest and thick gruel. Marcus, though, was not satisfied and ordered Galen to be sent for. Galen came but said and did nothing.

"Why do you remain silent?" Marcus enquired.

"These physicians who have been on campaign with you have had the better opportunity to make the correct diagnosis."

"Then, if you will do nothing else, take my pulse."

Galen did so.

"You have no fever," he declared, "merely an upset stomach."

"That's it! That's exactly it!" Marcus exclaimed. "I feel as though I'm weighed down by cold food."

"The usual remedy is peppered wine, but for an Emperor I would recommend also a pad of scarlet wool with ointment of nard applied to the anus."

"My own usual remedy." Marcus's stoic delight at this agreement was evident. "Pitholaus shall apply it."

When this was done, the Emperor had his feet massaged, ordered Sabine wine, sprinkled it with pepper and drank it.

From that day until his death four years on, Marcus always referred to Galen as "first among physicians and unique among philosophers".

But my joy at Marcus's recovery was short-lived. Panthea died. One moment I had been talking to her and the next she was dead. Galen was perplexed and could think of no explanation. As Marcus so gently said, "She has lain down to rest." Or, as my ancestors would have put it, "The gods have sent their messenger to fetch her."

In the few years – the very few years – we had been married, Panthea had made me sublimely happy. Happier in a way I had never experienced before. With an emotion approaching horror, I realized that my love for her had been a mortal love and that we would never again meet. It was a love unlike the love I had for Ishtar – that was immortal; however fleeting our encounters, I always knew that we would find each other again. But Panthea was gone for ever.

Marcus encouraged me to take a mistress, as he had done even though he regarded the sexual act as nothing more than "friction of the innards and convulsive ejaculation of mucus" – it was the comfort given to his spirit by intimate female company that mattered more. Yet I could not. I was inconsolable; I could not feel affection for any woman, still less endure physical contact.

A short while after Panthea's death, I came on Marcus meditating out loud. "Of human life," he was saying to himself, "time is a point, existence is a moving stream, sensation is dim, the whole fabric of the body susceptible to decay, fame uncertain – in brief, all things of the body are as a river, all things of the spirit a dream and a tomb; life is like a war and a sojourn in a foreign land. What then can set a man right? One thing and one alone: philosophy." I moved silently away, my presence undetected.

I wandered out of Rome, my footsteps aimless, hoping that Telesphorus would return from whatever adventure he had undertaken and discover me. Marcus Aurelius had enabled me to see that the love that outlasts the body is unattainable here on earth; human love may inspire mankind, but it is not to be trusted; in the end it is yet another illusion. Neither love nor woman shall be for me. I cannot bear the pain of their loss. My true love must be the love of medicine and its philosophy. Perhaps before his death Galen will have unravelled the tangled skein that it is. But in my heart I held little hope for, as I looked around and saw the hills of Rome slide into the mist, the words of Marcus returned to haunt me: "Look back at the past, how many changes of dynasties. You can foresee what is to come, for it will be of a totally similar pattern; it is impossible for it to escape the rhythm of the present. So, to study human life over forty years is the same as studying it over ten thousand."

8

*"If your faith is strong, God will be with you"**

If medicine were to be my true love, I was indeed chained to a fickle mistress whose present mood seemed set to plunge me into the depths of despair. After the death of Galen the path she trod led into the blackest of nights.

The Roman Empire was falling apart. The materialism of its ancient glory may have been maintained by an outward appearance of prosperity, but inwardly its temporal power was crumbling under the spiritual dominion of the Church of Rome. My mistress, too, was subject to that dominion though, held as she was, suspended between the worlds of reality and superstition, she simply bent with the wind. In one regard, however, her resilience was not enough: she became afflicted with an intense respect for the authority of the past which stifled her freedom of thought and prevented her from challenging her traditional beliefs – and any attempt she might have made earned a sharp rebuke.

Throughout my existence, the gods had been an intrinsic part of life. They may have squabbled among themselves but, as they had no spiritual or mystical baggage to encumber them, they were on the whole an astute down-to-earth assemblage with a generally reassuring effect on their mortal subjects.

In consequence, I was quite unprepared for the impact of monotheism. It was one thing to be brought up in the knowledge that there may be only one true God and to answer the call when it comes

*Early Christianity and medicine. *c.* 400 – *c.* 900. – J.G.

– as had the emperors of the now-divided Roman Empire. But it is quite another to have lived through three thousand years of polytheism and then to hear a man knock at your door saying: "Follow me". I found myself a stranger in a world whose values were, for me, an uncertain quantity. It was a world in which medicine was in confusion, having lost its sense of direction, and in danger of seeing its doctrines denied. But it was not just medicine, for the entire world was caught in a period of transition between two ages when events were governed by influences outside human control. Man had become aware of his individuality – as distinct from his being one of a tribe – and of his spirituality. He was to be in desperate need of help and guidance in the coming age though, as the ancient prophets had foretold, that help would be forthcoming – but would he make the best use of it?*

My footsteps were perhaps not as aimless as I had imagined for, two or three centuries beyond my leaving Rome, I was rejoined at Constantinople by Telesphorus.

"I was waiting for you." He greeted me as though we had parted yesterday which, with his manipulation of time, seemed the truth.

"Master, I did not ensure your arrival here for any good reason. Since yesterday," he gave one of his impish grins, "physicians have been in retreat from the understanding of medicine – such as it was – that Galen had reached. No one has been worth the hurrying of your footsteps. Indeed, I have only stopped you in Byzantium – I still cannot bring myself to call it Constantinople – as being a suitable place for you to take stock.

"Now come, I have gathered some books in your new home. They will give you an insight into the plight of medicine today." So saying, he took my hand and almost bounced along the marbled main street of the city before turning aside to lead me to a villa, secluded behind walls and a veritable forest of trees. Inside, all was prepared for me – the library was more than a mere gathering of books, it was a triumph of bibliological organization.

---

* Paul Baldassare is here speaking in astrological terms. The period of transition to which he refers is from the Age of Aries to that of Pisces at the beginning of the Christian era. As in all astrological periods of transition, new ideas were in conflict with the old; the existing pattern had to be discarded before the design of the new could be accomplished. Crises and uncertainties were inevitable. An "Age" in this context is a Great Month which lasts approximately two thousand, one hundred and sixty years. These Ages progress in the reverse direction to that of the more familiar Zodiacal constellations. – J.G.

"I have collected every...." Telesphorus caught my doubting look and began again. "I have collected copies of most of the books written since the death of Galen. I think you will find it instructive to compare them with Galen's own works – and I do have these in their entirety!" And he had – nearly four hundred of them in their varying lengths. There was work here to keep me pleasurably occupied for years.

I began with Galen, amusing myself by identifying the ideas and facts he had adapted from earlier writers; Telesphorus had thoughtfully acquired a score or more of the most important of these ancient works – he had spirited them away from the library in Alexandria when the city began its decline. That task completed I moved on to a study of the more recent volumes in chronological order (in obedience to Telesphorus's injunction!). I learnt nothing new; but what I did find of great interest was the manner in which Galen's work had been presented. He himself had been fairly discursive, not to say rambling, and this gave the later scholars an opportunity to bring together specific topics otherwise scattered throughout his writings. At first, speaking chronologically, these new books were straightforward copies of Galen, interspersed with excerpts from some of the pre-Galenic writers. But as time progressed, they began to omit Galen's philosophical musings and qualifications of his opinions. Instead they presented Galen as dogma. What was particularly disturbing was that this had destroyed Galen's sense of the unity of medicine and had led, in turn, to the separation of theory and practice, an error reinforced by a misunderstanding of Galen's teaching. Galen had indeed emphasized the importance of a philosophical approach to medicine – he either was, or wished to create the impression of being, a Stoic in the mould of Marcus Aurelius – but what he had not implied, as these later scholars had assumed, was that a physician had first to be educated as a philosopher.

In reading these travesties of Galen's writings, I was especially intrigued by a book of Magnus of Emesa that typified the extent to which these compilers would go. He had painstakingly worked his way through the entire Galenic corpus and extracted all the comments and observations on the urine. These he had put together as a handbook of the diagnosis of disease by uroscopy. [This book, Dr Annandale, had a greater influence than I suspected at the time. It marked the start of the study of the urine as an integral part of medical practice in the company of bloodletting and the study of the pulse. It even became a popular subject for artists of the Renaissance.]

During my years of study, I scarcely ventured into the city. Telesphorus saw to the management of the household and each day I walked in contemplative solitude in the grounds of the villa which were both extensive and beautiful with their sweeping views across the Bosporus. Sometimes I would wish for company, when Telesphorus would join me and we would pass the hours discussing my studies – usually in terms derogatory of the authors! At others, when I wished to hear a female voice, he would ensure that my walk was enlivened by a companion blessed with wit and physical attraction. We might bathe in the lake, but my emotions were never aroused – they had died long ago; my pleasures now came in the endless delight of my gardens throughout the ever-changing seasons.

My reading completed, Telesphorus and I were seated amidst the glories of a burgeoning land. Yesterday, the world had been shades of grey and black set against a turbulent sky; today the air had a new-found warmth and my garden was freshly green with touches of blue and gold, white and pink – order in disorder. It was the conviction that we were in the presence of my gods, the gods I knew and loved, that made me break the spell Nature had woven around us.

"Telesphorus, my friend, I am saddened by the story these books have to tell. The humoral foundations of our medicine may survive, though I fear Hippocrates would grieve at their condition. Yet the books are only scholars' work; they say nothing about healing in this new Christian world – and this, I know, is at odds with our understanding of disease. Because Galen, in his adherence to Aristotelian philosophy, wrote of a Creator who did nothing without a purpose, many Christians tolerate his ideas since these can be reconciled with their belief in the one God. For that, we must be thankful. And now, Telesphorus, as my work here is done, I shall return to Rome."

"Master, do not go. Your spirit will weep for the city; it is no longer the heart of a mighty empire. Stay here and you will find citizens of every race and from every country who will tell you what you wish to know. Go into the streets and ask!"

"No, Telesphorus. My mind is set. I must see for myself the consequences of this perplexing faith."

*   *   *

Telesphorus was right. I should never have returned to Rome. The city where my adored Panthea and I had wandered in the cool breezes of a summer evening lay in ruins, pillaged twice over. The only delight left for me to enjoy in the Forum was the profusion of wild flowers growing along the Via Sacra and amongst the fallen masonry strewn on every side. I scarcely felt surprise when I saw the Pantheon consecrated for Christian worship; but how Telesphorus's heart would have wept at this rejection of his family. I knew now why he had refused to accompany me.

I could find no one prepared to talk with me. As I quickly discovered, evidence of the influence of Christianity pervaded every aspect of medical life. Even to suggest that healing was a strictly medical preserve was to be condemned as a heretic. Had not Christ healed the sick by healing the soul, not the body? It was the soul that was all-important; the body was merely its temporary receptacle.

My mind was in turmoil. The comprehension of disease was no better than in the days of my ancestors and, in certain respects, could not even bear comparison with their ancient logic. For the thousand years since Hippocrates, medicine had been practised with some degree, at least, of practical rationality. But now all that had been swept away in the rising tide of spirituality. The responsibility for disease was laid elsewhere than on earth and, in consequence, its treatment had also to be sought in other realms.

The idea that disease was not sent by the gods but had a cause – whether identifiable or not – had been forgotten. The Christians believed that sickness was visited upon them as punishment for their sins and the sins of their fathers – a favoured site for the Lord's chastisement was the skin as this could be disfiguring and was there for all the world to see. Some fanatics even sought disease, sometimes by deliberate mortification of the flesh, as a test of their sanctity. When I questioned the Christians about their remedies, they could not deny that God had put healing medicines on earth, but they were there, they said, only for those whose faith was weak. "If your faith is strong, God will heal you" was a sentiment I often heard expressed. Yet I fear the faith of all too many was weak, as epidemics of "plague" [possibly bubonic plague this time, Dr Annandale, although malaria was rife in Italy] continued to ravage the Mediterranean lands carrying off great numbers of Christians and pagans alike.

Out in the countryside, remote from towns and cities, the Christian faith was less extreme and in places the Roman gods were still worshipped. The choice of healing practices was wide, but in the main relied, as it had for centuries, on folk medicine – as effective or as ineffective as it had ever been. I did, however, encounter the occasional physician who practised a diluted form of humoral medicine, though those of their patients who were Christians would usually follow the consultation with a visit to the nearest church or Christian shrine. When the patient was cured, the Church invariably claimed the credit for the miracle. God would heal, but only when He saw fit to do so. [Remission of chronic diseases, Dr Annandale, was regarded as a cure – and hence as a miracle. And, as I have said before, Nature is a wonderful healer of acute diseases if given a chance – another source of miracles.]

The longer I remained in what had been the Latin Empire, the more despondent I became. One day, Telesphorus, ever my watchful protector, appeared at my side.

"Bal-sarra-uzur, a new city has arisen beside the river Tigris in your own land. There, scholars of a new religion are working to preserve the old medicine. But before we leave I have something instructive to show you. You have already witnessed the baleful influence of the Christian church on medicine; now you shall see how the works of Hippocrates and Galen are being debased by so-say philosopher-physicians." And he led me to a public building where men were studying and talking around a large table. The books they were working on were those of Galen and were familiar to me. But they were not discussing their medical content. They were arguing about the meaning of the words. They believed that if they could interpret them correctly, the eternal truths of man's relationship with his God would be revealed to them. Quite how they came to this belief escaped me, as it did Telesphorus.

9

"Allah sends down no ailment without also sending down it for a cure" *

The desert air was cold. I pulled the burnous closer about me and shivered. I felt sick; the camel was the one mode of transport I loathed. I hated the uncertain-tempered vicious beasts. Beside me, quite at ease on his animal, Telesphorus kept up an incessant chatter to which I paid no attention as I was more concerned with complaining at my discomfort.

He had chosen, in his perversity, to restore my rapidly declining morale by making the final stage of our journey across apparently trackless desert.

"Bel-shazzar," he said, when we rested to eat before the day. "Marcus Aurelius showed you the nature of the true Stoic philosopher: a man of virtue** and above both pleasure and pain. But virtue cannot be learnt from books; it demands practice if it is to be sustained. And," a look more suited to a devil than an offspring of the gods came over his face, "and it has been many years since you suffered physical torment! Endure it as he would have endured it, in silence and without complaint."

Remembering, guiltily, what Marcus had said about pain: "what we cannot bear takes us away from life; what lasts can be borne", I resolved that Telesphorus should hear no more from me. Yet the train of thought

*Medicine in the world of Islam. c. 900 – 1037. – J.G.
** Here Telesphorus was using the word virtue in its ancient sense. "Virtus" was a Roman Republican concept – fearlessness in defence of one's male honour; courage; valour; integrity. It is almost impossible to translate adequately as it is, sadly, a concept that has lost its meaning today. – J.G.

he had started reawakened my memories of Panthea – these were a thing apart; they had nothing to do with Stoic philosophy, however admirable that might be; they were a part of my *mortal* life, they were the unbearable that had to be borne in this existence. I could not stem my tears.

"Why do you weep, Bal-sarra-uzur?"

"I weep for Panthea." My voice choked over her name. "Like all mortal beings she is gone, gone for ever."

"Master, have you still not divined the truth? When we met again in Byzantium I grieved with you. And whose words did I use to give you comfort?"

"You quoted something by Plato, but the words only eased my sadness; they did not reveal a mysterious truth."

"What I said might have been an epitaph for Panthea: 'You were the morning star among the living; and now you are the evening star giving new splendour to the dead.' My choice was inspired! But its message fell, as the Christians would say, on stony ground. Oh! Bal-sarra-uzur, do you forget that Ishtar is the morning and the evening star? In their infinite wisdom, the gods were setting you a trial. Unknown to you, Panthea was your beloved Ishtar sent into the world as a mortal for you to experience not only the beauty of mortal love but also the agony of its loss, believing it gone for ever."

I responded like a true mortal – with total incomprehension at the tricks the gods could play on us.

For day after day we rode on. Sometimes the sand was as smooth as silk, at others it rippled as if the ocean's waves had rested a moment before ebbing home. How I longed for those waves to cool the insufferable, the inescapable, heat. But, sitting on my accursed beast, aching in limbs and back, I kept my thoughts to myself; outwardly, at least, I was a good Stoic. Yet once when I lapsed into sleep and Telesphorus struck my animal into a gallop, I woke, screaming, from dreams of green valleys with cool, crystal waters flowing eternally in their depths; waters that had washed the dust and sand from my eyes, my ears, my mouth, my skin, my very soul.

After many days the desert changed and we passed through a mountainous land where the weather-worn rock towered high above in frantic shapes of brown and grey, where our voices came echoing back. Strange, perfectly formed pyramids that had never known the hand of man kept watch over the dead. What dead I know not, but dead they must have been for no man could live in this terrible world.

As we emerged from cliffs and precipices, the land grew more treacherous still. Leading our camels over smooth black stones shifting uncertainly beneath our feet we entered a wilderness where only the changing shape of the desert floor informed our progress from one area of burning wind-swept desolation to another.

"Telesphorus, how much further must we travel before we reach this newly-risen city?"

"We shall arrive at dawn, Bal-shazzar." I cursed him silently. This was his unvarying answer, and every time he nearly fell from his camel with laughter.

I reined back my beast and allowed Telesphorus to gain on me. Then I gave the animal its head to follow without my guidance. I looked up seeking inspiration, but in vain for the majestic beauty of the heavens was beyond my understanding. In the clear light of dawn the other worlds beyond our own began to disappear. Above us the sky was a vast unfathomable and endless void.

We must have been climbing steadily through the night, for we now found ourselves on a high rocky plateau. Instead of halting to rest through the heat of the day, Telesphorus continued riding. "We are nearly there, Master," he informed me, to my unutterable relief.

Before long we came to the edge of the heights and there in the far distance I could just discover the faint outline of a river with what looked to be a town on its banks. "That is Hit, Master, and the river is the Euphrates! From Hit, we shall take a boat down river to al-Anbar and from there travel the last few miles to Baghdad."

Only a Christian hermit brooding in the wilderness nurturing his immortal soul and dependent on passing travellers for sustenance until his body fell apart, could have been unaware of the changes that had taken place since the Prophet Mohamed had conquered Arabia in the name of Islam. In little more than a hundred years the Arab caliphs had extended his empire from Narbonne to Kabul in a mighty crescent through Spain, north Africa, Palestine, Syria, Mesopotamia, Armenia, Persia and Afghanistan to the Indus. The ancient Persian Empire had been destroyed and the Christian Eastern Roman Empire sat uneasily shrinking along the northern shores of the Mediterranean. The spiritual and cultural vitality of Islam was such that I forgave Telesphorus the nightmare of the journey. My morale was restored.

Nevertheless, with Christian Rome in mind, I reserved my personal judgment until I had gathered evidence of the influence of this new monotheistic religion on medicine. To this end, we travelled slowly and circuitously from al-Anbar, but I saw nothing to give me encouragement. Nothing differed in its essentials from anywhere else in the world outside the great cities. The people, poverty stricken as always, looked after themselves while those who could afford it resorted to a local healer or herbalist; the medicines were still governed by folklore and superstition. Indeed, so little had changed here since the days of my childhood that I felt like nothing so much as a mule condemned to circle the mill endlessly grinding the corn.

I had seen it all before. The jinn that brought disease were the very ones that had brought death to Ebih-Il. The charms to ward them off may not have been the statuettes of Abu; but no matter, if sickness struck the fault lay not with the belief but with the sick man's amulet or incantation which patently lacked the power to overcome the jinn. Disease was still regarded as a divine affliction; good health was the natural state of affairs. [I think, Dr Annandale, you will find the same principle applies in your world – perhaps with even greater force. The technological advances of your age have deluded people into the belief that good health should be theirs by *right* and if it is denied them, someone is to blame – not that far removed from my jinn? In fact, these advances should have persuaded them that reality is just the opposite.]

And so it was that I came to Baghdad, the capital city of the Abbasid caliphate. In the one hundred and fifty years since its foundation it had become the centre of the Islamic world and supported more than a million souls within its walls. I came as a physician from Alexandria because, even though, medically speaking, the city was but a faded shadow of its former greatness, it still preserved a reputation as a centre of Graeco-Roman medicine.

Telesphorus was insistent that unless I visited the Bayt al-Hikma, I would be a ship sailing through Islamic culture without a sight of the lodestar to navigate by.

He was right, of course. The Bayt al-Hikma was a worthy successor to Ptolemy's universal library in Alexandria and the true cultural heart of a great empire. In the years since Caliph al-Ma'mun had transformed an idea into a building, travellers had returned with books and medicines from Persia, India and as far afield as China, and scholars had been despatched to discover missing texts. And to preserve the accumulating wisdom within Islamic culture, all was translated into Arabic.*

From the manner of their dress, however, I saw that many of the translators were Christians.

"The language of these Christians is Syriac," Telesphorus answered my question. "You have lived too long under the mantle of Christianity to understand why the world of Islam welcomes men of other faiths and of all countries who bring with them their scholarship. Islam seeks knowledge, whatever its source. It was through intolerance that the Christian world descended into the cultural abyss."

"Nevertheless," – it did Telesphorus no harm to be contradicted once in a while – "it is the scholarship of the Christians that enables Islam to save the ancient knowledge!"

The full extent of that scholarship became evident when I began to study the Arabic texts. These were not literal, unthinking translations of the Greek but carefully considered expressions of the sense of the originals, most of which were liberally bespattered with abstruse philosophical commentaries. This was essential if the Arab scholars – highly intelligent men, fluent in Greek, Arabic and Syriac (a sort of half-way house between the other two) – were to grasp the fundamental nature of Greek science.

As I read on, I noticed that passages in the original Greek were missing from the translations. I drew this to the attention of Qusta ibn Luqa, a Christian. He was an old man and seemed surprised not only at my having identified the missing sections, but also that I, to all appearances a devout Moslem, should question their omission.

"Bel-shazzar," his voice was soft and, after speaking my name, he continued in Greek. "*You* should know that the passages we omit are offensive to the religion of Islam. But since the Koran contains few allusions to medicine, the problems for us are also few and we are able

* In this section of his story, Paul Baldassare is inconsistent in his use of names. Sometimes he gives them in Arabic (using the English alphabet), sometimes in full and sometimes in its shorter form. In doing so, he would seem to follow "the old fashion of writing the best phonetic approximation according to ordinary English spelling" – as A.W. Lawrence said of his brother's (T.E.'s) practice in *Seven Pillars of Wisdom*. Mostly, though, he is inclined to use the form most familiar in the West. – J.G.

to construct a seamless text so that only..." here he paused and looked at me in the way I had come to recognize. He was one of those intuitively perceptive people who, given in their cup those last few drops of divine understanding, could have read my history, "...only an exceptional scholar would appreciate their absence."

I reassured him that I was not prying into his work which, indeed, he knew I admired, but wished merely to learn whether the scholarship of the Bayt al-Hikma had filtered beyond its walls.

"When I first came here more than forty years ago," he replied, "the answer would have been very little. The traffic in books was all inwards and our responsibility was to make the knowledge accessible to scholars. But it was a time of transition when the flow both of untranslated books and, alas! of our income began to evaporate like the dew in the morning sun. My master, Hunayn ibn Ishaq, a Nestorian priest and the greatest scholar I have known, realized that unless we continued our studies in a new form, the work of the Bayt al-Hikma – at least insofar as medicine was concerned – would ossify and die and be lost to Islam. In his later years, he completed many texts that were deficient either on account of loss or of the original author's failure, whether from ignorance or simple abandonment, to complete the work. Before he died he wrote an original treatise on the eye which has been much read by physicians.

"I continued in his ways but I have also trodden paths other than those of medicine. I have explored the sciences of astronomy, physics and mathematics and I have written new works which extend the understanding of these subjects." Suddenly Qusta ibn Luqa stopped, conscious that a lack of modesty might seem discourteous.

I urged him to continue. All knowledge, I said, was welcome to me and when it was given me by its originator, it was doubly so.

"When a man has absorbed himself as deeply as did Hunayn and as have I in the writings of others, he is often permitted to discern an inner meaning that perhaps eluded the original writer. We are then able to build upon these revelations.

"Galen remains the authority and because he provides evidence for a divine Creator who determines the order of nature, his work is unquestioningly accepted by the followers of Islam – as it is by those of Christ – and his teachings on humoral medicine are the practice of physicians in the cities of the Empire. At one time, the philosophies of the East, of India and Persia, were popular, but they fell from favour, though some aspects, such as the Indian system of numerals, have persisted."

Qusta ibn Luqa had been studying me intently with a view, I thought, to discovering how far he could trust me. Then, without warning, he changed the subject, coming straight to his point without any of the customary preliminaries.

"You are not an Arab. I doubt you are even a Believer," he began. I said nothing. "Your features are not Arabic, although I cannot define their origins. But with your eyes, it would not surprise me to learn that you came from another world!" He smiled, knowing full well I would neither deny nor confirm his suspicions.

"The name, Bayt al-Hikma is translated into Greek and other non-Semitic tongues as 'House of Wisdom'." Where, I wondered was this leading? I was having difficulty following his train of thought. "But I see you know this already. What you may not know is that, in principle, the wisdom of Islam coincides with the wisdom of the Greeks. It signifies the search for truth wherever it may be found: that which is true is Islamic. [Do not, Dr Annandale, confuse this with: *only* that which is Islamic is true.] It thus lies within the same conceptual stream as the old Arab tradition which maintains that when a number of possibilities exist, only one can be the absolute truth – though it may, nevertheless, be expressed in a number of different ways – while all the others are absolutely false.

"Medicine's truths are still hidden and, to my mind, none will ever be considered absolute. Both Islam and my own religion stand astride the path that leads towards the understanding of disease" – I saw now why he had been debating whether or not to trust me – "and even were they to be removed, I fear the path would prove endless."

Resigned though I was to an acceptance of this same fear, it still distressed me to hear it expressed by a mortal. I turned to look at I know not what to hide my tears.

"There is a sect, the Ikhwan al-Safa," he was saying when I had calmed my emotion and was able to look at him again, "who believe that the study of man's anatomy and physiology holds the key to the wisdom and power of God the Creator. They have established – to their own satisfaction – a correspondence between the anatomy of the human body and the anatomy of the heavens; this, they achieved by means of a numerical symbolism, not by anatomical study.

"I am torn apart like a liver the dogs have been at. I do not know what I believe." It was a long time since I had encountered a man of such intellectual honesty. "I am a Christian. I work with the followers of the Prophet so that the writings of ancient Graeco-Roman scholars may become known to them. And yet I cannot see where it will lead. We are bound by the chains of faith. The Koran proscribes the dissection of the human body – as does Christianity. Animals may be dissected, but I am not alone in thinking that the animal anatomy cannot be equated with that of man. Both faiths believe the dead feel pain; and we are agreed that on the Day of Judgement we shall all be summoned before the throne of God to account for the sufferings of the body He has given into our charge. There can be no escape; any desecration of His gift will be there for all to witness. I believe in Christ, but I cannot believe that a loving God would condemn a man to eternal damnation for the loss of an arm in battle or of a limb amputated by a surgeon to save his life. Neither can I believe that a man whose dismembered body was carried before God should also be condemned because another was seeking to understand His miraculous work."

Later, thinking on his words, I wondered how his Christian contemporaries had reconciled their beliefs with the embracing of martyrdom by their early predecessors – a fate that could entail beheading, mutilation in gladiatorial combat and much else besides. Alas! I was denied the opportunity of debating the question with him.

When I next visited the Bayt al-Hikam, Qusta ibn Luqa was dead. His departure from this world coincided with the spread of Arabic learning throughout the Empire, most notably to the Western Caliphate in Spain. Books, texts and manuscripts in Arabic made their way to distant lands by the very trade routes along which they had arrived centuries earlier in their original languages.

If Qusta ibn Luqa had been inclined to despair for the future, maybe because he viewed the world through his books, the Persian physician Rhazes was fashioned from a mould of a very different design. Although he, too, was widely read and had an exemplary respect for past authority, his first words to me were completely unexpected:

"All that is written in books is worth much less than the experience of a wise physician." My heart warmed to him. Besides, he was one of the kindest of men and his lined old face lit up with a smile as he spoke. Had he not given freely of his time and skill to the more unfortunate of his patients, he could have been the wealthiest of the wealthy physicians of Baghdad.

"We are few, Bel-shazzar, and the sick are many. If we cannot help them directly, we must help them to help themselves." He handed me a book from a little pile at his side; it was *Man la yahduruhu al-tabib**. "In this I have written down many prescriptions which the poor may have prepared for them. Nevertheless, when a man's health is disturbed, he should first look to his diet before having recourse to drugs – and these should always be as simple as circumstances permit."

I was not surprised at this last caveat since pharmacy and chemistry had become sciences in their own right in the melting-pot of Islamic culture. Treatments were moving rapidly beyond the simple, though numerous, herbals of Dioscorides. When I saw such practices as sublimation, calcination, crystallization and distillation and heard the chemists describe their preparations as alkalis, alcohols, syrups, elixirs and many other strange terms, I had a peculiar (and, I have to admit, not very pleasant) feeling that physicians might be able to cure diseases before they understood them.

We were seated in the large central courtyard of the hospital in Baghdad of which Rhazes was physician-in-charge. The scattered few Christian hospitals I had visited in the West bore no comparison with this magnificent institution. The courtyard was a beautifully laid-out garden with fountains gently playing and trees offering a welcome shade to plants and patients alike.

"We Moslems," – since my encounter with Qusta ibn Luqa I had made no attempt to appear a Moslem. I was simply a Greek physician from Alexandria with no identifiable beliefs. "We Moslem physicians," he repeated, "regard the body to be an extension of the soul. Illnesses that manifest themselves in the body may thus not be of the body itself but of the soul: to heal the body, we must heal the soul. In this we differ from the Christian belief which holds the body in little regard – it is only the temporary abode of the soul." He paused and looked me, wondering whether, in saying this he might have offended me. But I reminded him that my religious beliefs were not strong and did, in any case, take second place to my curiosity to learn about medical practice

* *Who has no Physician to attend him. –* J.G.

in the countries I travelled through.

He handed me another book from his little pile.

"This also I have written. Please accept it as a gift. I think the subject will be new to you. I have entitled it *Spiritual Physick* and in it you will read how, in treating disease arising in the soul, we value most highly music, beautiful scenery and agreeable companionship. Such a receipt is balm to the troubled spirit." [This, Dr Annandale, was the beginning of what you now know as psychological and psychosomatic medicine.]

"Forgive me, Bel-shazzar, if I must leave you. I have patients to attend to and students to teach." He rose, gathered up his books and walked slowly across the courtyard into the hospital building.

Rhazes must have been as anxious to talk to me as I was to learn from him. On the next day as I was sitting on the same seat, he walked out of the building and when his attention was drawn to my presence, he went out of his way to join me. We greeted each other warmly.

"You study and practise the medicine of Hippocrates and Galen?" I questioned him. He bowed his head in acknowledgement.

"But is this not in disagreement with Arab-Islamic medicine?"

"Not at all! Not at all! Both believe that men should keep in good health. Where we differ is in our beliefs about the cause of disease. Hippocrates maintained that diseases were natural events with natural causes, but we believe – as do the Christians on this occasion – that disease is a punishment for sin. We also believe it possible that some diseases, perhaps those that arise in the spirit, are sent by the jinn. Where we diverge from the Christians is in attaching no stigma to disease. The Prophet has said, 'Allah sends down no ailment without also sending down for it a cure.' So our task is to seek out, with divine help, the cure that Allah has provided.

"But for those who wish to entrust themselves entirely to Allah rather than relying on a physician such as myself as intermediary, there is the *Medicine of the Prophet*. This is a compilation of writings derived from all manner of sources. It began life as a collection of questions on medical matters posed to the Prophet during his lifetime and the answers he gave, as recalled by his followers. As the years passed, it grew to contain anecdotes, aphorisms, folklore, religious dicta and purely common-sense advice. Even aspects of humoral medicine are recommended."

It was some years before we next sat together in that enchanted courtyard, by which time Rhazes's faltering sight had almost completely deserted him. Rumour had it that the failure had started after a brutal beating at the hands of the caliph in punishment for his outspokenness, but he maintained it was simply a matter of advancing years and his intense preoccupation with writing. He had composed more than two hundred works on subjects ranging from alchemy to ethics and from anatomy and physiology (much of which, in view of the proscription on dissection, was an arrangement of earlier writings) to medicine, surgery, obstetrics and beyond.

I suggested I might act as his amanuensis, an offer he readily accepted. Throughout his life he had recorded the smallest detail of every patient he had treated and had insisted that similar notes were kept in his hospital. On his death, I collected all his own notes – which, besides the details of the patients, contained his comments and apposite quotations from other books – and did my best to arrange them in a manageable order. Although I knew they had been for his private use, I took steps to ensure they were made available to all who asked. I called them his *Al-Hawi fi l-tibb**.

[I realize, Dr Annandale, that my attempts at achieving manageability would not have met with modern approval. Ignorance of disease states made any form of organization or classification difficult, if not impossible. Nevertheless, Rhazes's descriptions of smallpox and measles are, unlike so many ancient case histories, instantly recognizable.]

*   *   *

The last, so it transpired, of the great Arabic physician-compilers, Avicenna by name, had been my friend – though not Telesphorus's – since the days of his precocious youth. His intellect was formidable. As a boy, he had outstripped his teachers; he had mastered the Koran at the age of ten; and at twenty-one he had written an encyclopaedia of science. No facet of human knowledge escaped his attention and he was greatly sought after for his legal and political opinions. But it was medicine and philosophy that took pride of place. His weakness was an inability to resist a pretty face and, not for the first time, he had become involved in an intrigue at court. On this occasion, the lady

---

* *The All-Inclusive Work on Medicine*. This massive compendium was later (thirteenth century) translated into Latin as the *Continens*. – J.G.

had a high-ranking protector and Avicenna had had to flee for his life. Yet his misfortune was my gain. Until the dust had settled over Isfahan, he sought refuge in my house.

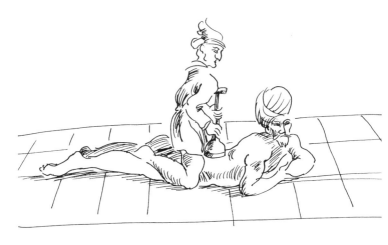

Treating a spinal condition, as illustrated in Avicenna's Canon.

He spent much of his time with me in my library working on his *Canon of Medicine*. In writing this, he based his philosophy on Aristotle and his medicine on Galen, blending the two into a unity that was unmistakably his own. From the practical point of view, his great achievement was his revision of Galen's writings. This he was able to do in a way that had been impossible for the previous commentators whose work I had so admired all those years ago in Constantinople. The *Canon* contained for the first time, an organized, systematic statement of medical knowledge – adorned with Avicenna's own opinions!* On one point, however, I was not so sure I agreed with him; this was his insistence on separating surgery from medicine.

"I have seen," he said, "many a good physician who was unable to use a knife as it should be used. A surgeon should, perhaps, be a good physician but a good physician need not be a good surgeon. The talents

*The eighteenth-century Swiss physiologist, Albrecht von Haller (1708 – 1777) called the *Canon* a "methodical inanity"! – J.G.

required for each are different."

I still had my doubts.

"In our country*," he continued, "I would recommend the use of the cautery rather than the knife. Wounds heal more favourably in our dry and dusty climate." With this I was inclined to agree.

Before he left my house to return to the court at Isfahan – with a pardon – he made an intriguing observation:

"Conflicts are sometimes not without their benefits. The friction between Islam and Christianity over the possibility that some diseases may be contagious, has drawn physicians together to defend the concept. We now accept that it is true!"

When he had gone Telesphorus, who was glad to see the back of him, remarked: "That man, for all his intelligence, is a rogue." I raised my eyebrows at him. "He is not long for this life. His delight in savouring the pleasures of this world and his obsession with his own intellectual brilliance will bring him to an early grave. But, Master, I ask you how many sick people has he treated? How much of his surgical writings are pure book-learning?"

[I do not know why Telesphorus adopted this stance, though I suspect he may have been jealous of his Greek heritage and was displeased at seeing it usurped, even if only indirectly. On the other hand, it may have been that his long association with a mortal had inculcated in him some of our irrational prejudices! However, despite Telesphorus's scepticism, Dr Annandale, there can be no doubting Avicenna's lasting influence. His *Canon* was still a part of the curriculum in Egypt in the late nineteenth century. And, as another instance of the resilience of Islamic medicine, you are quite likely to find copies of the *Medicine of the Prophet* on the bookshelves of Islamic households today.]

*Avicenna was born in Bukhara in what is now Uzbekistan. – J.G.

10

Medicine - An exercise in the art of translation*

y humours were in sore disarray. An intellectual movement** sweeping through Christendom appeared set to clarify some aspects, at least, of the nature of disease; but as it took shape I saw it to be no more than a sham, an embellishment of the abstruse and interminable arguments that had so preoccupied philosophers in past centuries. The question now uppermost in men's minds was how to apply the logic of Aristotle to an understanding, not of man and disease, but of the Christian God – illogically, or so it seemed to me, medicine was ignored. When, in a very few centres, it did manage to creep into the curriculum the purpose was not to produce trained physicians but to delve deeper into the relationship between man and God, his Creator.

I was now more convinced than ever that each time man turned a corner in his history or ventured along an untrodden path, he divested himself of some hard-earned fragment of medical knowledge, leaving it to rot in the mire. Fortune smiled only when a scholar passed along the way in later years and rescued the fragment before its message became obliterated for all time.

Since leaving Baghdad my wanderings had once more been utterly aimless and Telesphorus must have found me a sour companion. But while I was continually morose and consumed by misery, he was

*The Middle Ages. c. 1037 – c. 1330. J.G.
** Scholasticism. This flourished between the 12th (some say the 9th) and early 15th centuries. The Scholastics rediscovered Arabic, and through them, Aristotelian philosophies. – J.G.

126

unfailingly cheerful in his search for the plans devised by the gods for the benefit – or otherwise – of mankind.

"Master, you know you cannot influence Nature's great design," he spoke with sympathy for my plight as we made our way between Arles and Aix in the spring of the year. "Remember Rhazes, and when your soul is sick, seek the healing balm of serenity in all that is beautiful around you."

But even the scent of that most beautiful of lands could not ease my burden.

"My mistress has deserted me and you ask me to seek peace in beauty!" My words came more sharply than I intended and I was relieved when Telesphorus took no offence. Indeed, I doubt that he noticed, so eager was he to chide me for my faults.

"Balthasar, are you both blind and deaf?" He had me by the hand and pulled me round to face him; his strength never ceased to surprise me. "You have stubbornly refused to make a home in France, rather you have chosen to walk – to walk! not even to ride like the nobleman you are! – from town to town in the hope of meeting another Galen, another Hippocrates. No, Balthasar! such hopes are forlorn if you insist on walking with your eyes shuttered and your ears blocked – they are forlorn anyway," he muttered under his breath but just loud enough for me to hear. "You must look at people to see where they come from. You must talk to them to learn what they have to say.

"In your search for a king you have ignored the peasant. Have you been completely oblivious of the physicians who come to France after studying in the south of Italy? They have learnt from ancient commentaries on Galen and, for the most part, are good practical exponents of the art."

I looked blankly at him. "Where have they studied?" I asked in disbelief.

"Salerno. There, there is a school where the monks have studied at the excellent library of Monte Cassino."

"Then we must go to Salerno!" In the twinkling of an eye my vitality returned; my mistress was restored to me and I could not act quickly enough. I sent Telesphorus to buy the best horses the district could offer and away we went. I was borne by a Pegasus of the new millennium.

The old Roman health resort of Salerno was not greatly impressive and its school, in size, could not compare with the intellectual emporia

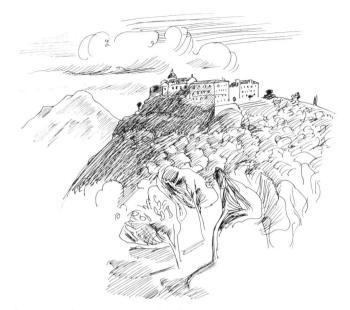

The monastery of Monte Cassino. Secure from the worldly exchanges far below them, the monks pursued their labours in uninterrupted calm.

of France. Where it excelled was in cultural vibrancy. And nowhere else in the world were healers taught in the same manner. When I questioned the monks about the source of their knowledge, the name that kept recurring was Constantinus – called Africanus since he came from Tunisia. And where might I find him? I asked. At Monte Cassino, where he had recently retired to continue his literary work.

Perched high on a precipitous mountain top, the monastery of Monte Cassino had been designed on the lines of an impregnable fortress. Secure from the worldly exchanges far below them, the monks pursued their labours in uninterrupted calm.

Telesphorus insisted that he came with me when I visited Constantinus in his cell. The reason, he said, was to meet the man and learn from him, but in reality it was to prepare himself for my reaction to what I was about to discover. Surrounded by books, Constantinus was solemnly translating Galen, Hippocrates and their Arabic commentators into Latin. It was unbelievable! I had been through all this before; it was as if medicine was merely an exercise in the art of translation. Somehow I managed to retain a civil tongue in my head and discuss intelligently some obscure Hippocratic argument – much to the amazement of Constantinus.

"Telesphorus, this is absurd! We are no further forward than when Galen was alive – and he has been dead now some eight hundred years." I was furious with Telesphorus, with Constantinus, with Salerno, with the entire world and everything on it.

"Am I to believe that an understanding of disease will come only when Galen and Hippocrates have been translated into every tongue at Babel? That cannot be so, and foolish also is the man who thinks it can be reached through philosophy alone!"

"Oh, Balthasar, Balthasar!" Telesphorus was grinning with delight. "Anger sits better on you than misery. The monk wishes to talk with you again tomorrow – his work goes beyond translation and I think you will approve of his achievements."

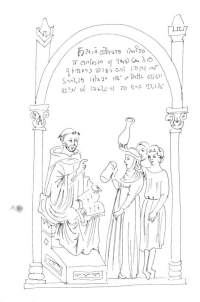

Constantinus Africanus lecturing on uroscopy.

I had my doubts, but the next day we returned to Constantinus's cell. As our conversation proceeded, it was soon apparent that Telesphorus's forecast had been correct.

"Galen's writings were obscure and confused," Constantinus began. "The commentaries of later writers sometimes clarified an argument, but more often added to the confusion. It requires a very perceptive mind to unravel Galen's reasoning. When his texts were translated into Arabic, not only did they encounter a new language but also an alien culture and a new style of thought. Consequently the translators were compelled to reinterpret Galen's ideas and most did so with remarkable competence." (I chose to overlook the man's remarkable condescension!)

"Now it has become our turn to make the true medicine of the ancients accessible to our students by translating the Arabic texts into Latin. We have allowed ourselves more licence than those who made the Arabic translations as our culture is more advanced and we have a few hundred years more learning to draw on. We have, you might say, 'opened up' Galen to an extent that has been impossible hitherto.

"To show you what I mean, this is a translation I have prepared of Johannicius's *Questions on Medicine*."

Constantinus handed me a book entitled *Liber ysagogarum*. I looked at it and then at him; I was totally perplexed.

"Are you perhaps an Arabic scholar yourself?" he asked.

When I answered that I was, he picked up an old book from among those lying on a table.

"You recognize it now, I see." He could hardly have missed my expression as I found myself given a copy of Hunayn ibn Ishaq's *Al-Masa'il fi l-tibb**.

"We know Hunayn as Johannicius but, by whatever name, his writings hold the key to the understanding of Galen. So, after passing through a Nestorian Christian, a Tunisian monk and several hundred years (an inconsequentiality to the Lord) Galen's work has come alive, and the essence of his philosophy can at last be given practical expression.

"As you are a physician familiar with the old concepts of Hippocratic and Galenic medicine, this new understanding will be of value to you

* *Questions of Medicine*. – J.G.

130

and, moreover, you will be able to spread the knowledge on your travels."

In the next hour my eyes and ears were opened and many obscurities that had plagued me over the centuries were cleared away. Constantinus was an excellent teacher*.

First, he explained how, as time went on, the Hippocratic waters had become muddied and even Galen had failed to clear them. "Now, through Johannicius, I have reached the truth.

"Good health is wholly in the power of six orders of what I have termed non-naturals: the sleeping and the waking states; movement and repose; food and drink; fullness and excretion; and finally the passions and the emotions. If these non-naturals do not receive their due attention, the body grows sick. A consideration of imminent changes in the needs of the body – whether on account of changes in climate, forthcoming exertion and the like – allows a man to adjust the non-naturals and so prevent a disruption of the humours."

[This interpretation of Galen's philosophy, Dr Annandale, led in the coming centuries to countless books of advice on how to restore and preserve health. Although many of these appeared, at first glance, to deal only with diet, this was not the case. To the authors, the word "diet" referred to a person's entire way of life.]

*   *   *

Despite Constantinus's insight into the works of Galen, I remained unaware of any progress in the understanding of disease that could be put to practical use. The poor still suffered from diseases their folk-healers were unable to cure, and the rich still endured the ministrations of their physicians who only added to the sufferings of disease.

Universities and hospitals sprang up across Europe and, as they were founded, I enrolled in one university after another, but invariably I was one of a mere handful of students studying medicine. At every one we were subjected to the same Aristotelian philosophy of the logical progression from universal causes to specific effects. We were taught how matter was created, how it was changed, and how it obeyed the universal laws. From this we were supposed to see how it applied to

---

* Dr Baldassare's enthusiasm for the work of Constantine the African is not shared by all recent medical historians, though most agree that his translations had a lasting influence. Typical of the criticisms are that his translations of the Arabic texts were inaccurate and rendered into bad Latin, and that his knowledge of medicine was negligible. But he evidently impressed Dr Baldassare! (The charge of bad Latin has also been levelled at many other translators of this era.) – J.G.

mankind. [Every generation has to make use, as best it can, of the information available to it. Your data, Dr Annandale, sometimes prove wide of the mark – and who knows how much more will prove false in years to come?]

The Christian Church had shifted its ground and now believed that at the Day of Judgement all mankind would stand before the throne of God, where those who had been mutilated or become dust and ashes would be made whole again. Whether this was its motivation or not, the Church had sanctioned dissections – provided the body was that of a executed felon and his remains given a decent Christian burial. Even so, dissections were occasional affairs – once a month, once a year or less, maybe – attended with considerable pomp and ceremony, and of more religious than medical benefit.

These anatomies were presided over by the Magister, resplendent in his doctoral robes and seated above the proceedings on an often ornately carved canopied throne. He was attended by a prosector and a medical student, also in academic dress. The student's duty was to read from the Magister's favourite anatomical text to indicate to the prosector what he was supposed to be exposing. Rather than explain the different organs and structures in anatomical terms, the Magister, in his commentaries, related them to the philosophy of Galen and the one Creator – thus the "truths" revealed were acceptable to the Christian Church.

When I was attending the more secularly inclined university at Padua we once had the unusual experience of having a female corpse for dissection. This attracted a large audience of fifty or more citizens anxious to discover the mysteries of the female body. The Magister (whose name I forget) decided that I should read the anatomical text. His chosen authority was Aretaeus (almost a contemporary of Galen!) who, in his opinion, was the greatest physician since Hippocrates. The demonstration took place in a church and as soon as the Magister was enthroned, I began:

"In the middle of the flanks of women lies the womb, a female viscus, closely resembling an animal; for it is moved of itself hither and thither in the flanks, also upwards in a direct line to below the cartilage of the thorax, and also obliquely to the right or left, either to the liver or spleen; and it likewise is subjected to prolapsus downwards, and, in a word, it is altogether erratic."

As I recited in solemn, measured tones pausing, when I caught his eye, to allow the Magister to deliver a commentary, the prosector manhandled the uterus in a vain attempt to demonstrate its supposed motions.

"It delights also," I continued, "in fragrant smells, and advances towards them; and it has an aversion to foetid smells, and flees from them; and on the whole, the womb is like an animal within an animal."

For three days this highly imaginative litany continued. At the start, only those standing closest could have caught sight of the organs as they were displayed and by the end even the prosector was unable to define the putrefying muscles. If nothing else, here was proof indeed that the human body was but the temporary residence of man's immortal soul!

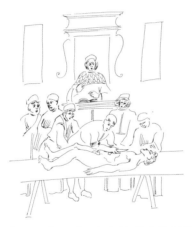

Mondino, seated above the proceedings and resplendent in his doctoral robes, presides over an anatomy.

To describe most of these anatomies as farcical would be to do them greater justice than they deserved, though a notable exception were those of Mondino de Luzzi. He employed, as assistant prosector, Alessandra Gilliani who, to the amazement of all, had the skill to dissect out the blood vessels to their smallest divisions without damage. She then prepared them for Mondino's demonstration by filling them with coloured liquids that hardened, allowing her to paint the arteries and veins in their natural colours.

In Spain, they were still translating as if the future of the world depended on it. Over the years, though, I had met a handful of Spanish physicians – Christians, Moors, Jews, alike – who achieved recognition through their writings; the Arabic influence was, not unexpectedly, predominant. Their scholarship was of a high level and they continued to bring yet more order and a deeper comprehension to the ancient

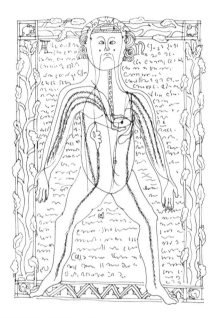

Thirteenth century concept of the cardiovascular system. From a mediaeval manuscript.

works than had previous translators. In this sense medicine was moving forward. But in the treatment and understanding of disease, in the healing of the sick, there was little change. In the Christian world, much compassion was extended to the poor in the monasteries and in the hospitals (which, for the most part, were run by religious orders anyway), but this was for the good of their eternal souls rather than the comfort of their suffering bodies.

The one faint glimpse of encouragement was the appearance of works translated into the vernacular. These were mainly surgical treatises –

as if to drive home the widening gulf between the "academic" discipline of medicine and the despised barbarity that was surgery. Even so, the books that circulated frequently described the most intricate operations; their wealth of beautifully drawn instruments reminded me of those with which Avicenna had decorated his books – though not, if Telesphorus was correct, employed on patients. Regrettably, reality was not reflected in their pages. Few operations were performed and happy the patient who did not journey to oblivion on a tide of his own blood or endure the lingering agony of a festering death.

"Telesphorus," I said, "I have reached a moment of decision. For how many centuries have we travelled together and for how many more did I travel alone before you came to me as a companion beyond imagined worth?" Dear Telesphorus, I truly loved him and he was not averse to occasional flattery – even though he was never quite sure how to react.

"Telesphorus," I continued, "there is nothing but night along this endless road named Medicine. The straight and ancient road from Greece and Rome is now a rutted, dusty, treacherous track. What is medicine now?" I asked, rhetorically. "It is yet another illusion. It is no more than a magic sleight of hand." I paused waiting for him to accuse me of inconsistency, but he remained silent. Anger and frustration were rising within me. "All the innumerable books – most of them of interminable length and full of false philosophy – have for centuries been merely the amulets, charms and incantations of the 'learned' physician! They might as well wear them around their necks as read them for all the good they do the sick!" I had never been so venomously inclined towards my brother practitioners.

"I have lost all hope. At the next turning I shall strike out along a different path in search of understanding."

"Yes, Master," was his only response. He refused to discuss my intention. His unspoken disapproval was so vehement that I should have heeded it. I did not. I blundered on, stubbornly believing I was in the right; that I would find the understanding of disease along a different route.

11

The Black Death ensures that life will never be the same again*

iammetta kissed me.

"For, as the last degree of joy brings with it sorrow, so misery has ever its sequel of happiness." Giovanni Boccaccio would have been pleased that I should borrow his words, even though he was now victim to the former state while I rejoiced in the latter. He knew I had not stolen Fiammetta from him – their ways had parted some months before our chance encounter in the square of San Lorenzo. Our eyes had responded and, with hands clasped, we had climbed the steps into the church. There, in the cool midday twilight lit only by the candles of the penitents, Fiammetta kissed me.

Her lips brushed mine with the gentleness of an angel's wing and in that instant my ancient resolve never again to fall under the spell of mortal woman was doomed like the flame of a shattered lamp. Yet Paradise lay not in her kiss, nor in her eyes that wakened untold and long-forgotten passions. No, Paradise dwelt deep in her heart, in her innocent kindness – the innocence that delights in every living thing and the kindness that is beyond wisdom.

Powerless to resist, I had been drawn back to Naples from Spain in the certain knowledge that I was again to find Ishtar alive. Telesphorus, however, had declined to accompany me.

"If you wish to believe that understanding lies in strange places, you will discover only falsehoods." He was still resentful and not to be

*Boccaccio describes the effects of the plague. c. 1330 – 1348. – J.G.

136

placated. Nevertheless, he gave the distinct impression that, had he wished, he could have explained the fixation with the ancients that so disturbed me. On the morning of my departure, I decided to confront him.

"You know why medicine remains chained to the past, yet you refuse to tell me. Why?" I demanded.

"The time has not yet come." He was taking delight in infuriating me. "You see only the outward signs of the philosophers' thoughts while their profound concerns lie beyond your present comprehension." At that moment I could have dismembered him. "But Balthasar, be patient." He saw that I was in no mood for his goading, however playfully intended, and laid a sympathetic hand on my arm.

"Master, if I was permitted to open your eyes to the future, even for the briefest moment, I would willingly do so. But you are mortal – an unusual example, I admit," he giggled. "And so you must endure the uncertainties of a mortal's existence.

"Farewell! and do not forget that the real treasures of the world you inhabit arrive unannounced and in the most unexpected places." And with that typically enigmatic remark he slapped the hindquarters of my horse and I was off like the wind for Naples. "But you will not find the understanding you seek where you are going." His final words reached my ears as faintly as a receding echo.

In that first moment in the church of San Lorenzo, all memory of the past was expelled from my mind. The centre of my universe was Fiammetta – I could no more think of her as Maria as I could believe the Vicar of Christ had converted to Islam; if Boccaccio's mistress was now mine, why should I feel shame at loving her by the name he had given her?

I had long known that the deliberate pursuit of happiness was always destined to fail even before the chase had begun. But happiness came with Fiammetta at the dawn of each new day. To be loved by this most beautiful of creatures was Paradise enough. When drawn apart by necessity, I sank into misery until I could hear her voice on the gentle breeze singing softly "I love you".

When we had quite exhausted the pleasures of Naples, we journeyed leisurely northwards through her father's kingdom and on into the Papal States until at length we came to Assisi. Hitherto, we had been royally entertained in castle and villa and escorted on by the host's mounted guard. Our road had been determined by Fiammetta's delight in the sanctity of the multitude of churches and abbeys that dominated the landscape. Even greater was the inner peace she drew from contemplation of the paintings ornamenting every last space within these temples – which I sensed were witness more to the vanity of man than the glory of God. Although Fiammetta worshipped as a good Christian, I was never sure how deep lay her religious convictions; yet her life would have adorned any faith or any world motivated by love and an open heart.

Her chosen destination was Assisi, but before we entered the town, she dismissed our servants and retainers, telling them to find lodgings until we should be ready to leave. Then, taking me by the hand, she led me through the woods to the Porziuncola.* There we spent the night on our knees praying, each in our own way. There, too, I think I was as close to the Christian God as I had ever come, or was ever likely to come again. But my prayers were haunted by the Saint's dying verses recorded in his *Canticle of the Creatures:* "Praise to you, my Lord, for our sister Death, for no one living can escape her." I wept at the irony of these words.

The next morning we roused ourselves – for we had both slumbered during our vigil – and walked the league** into town. Rising before us, in complete contrast to the humble Porziuncola, was the monumental fortress of the double basilica dedicated to St Francis – not that such an edifice would have found the remotest flicker of favour with the Saint who, both by word and example, had preached the gospel of Holy Poverty. His spirit had even to endure the "ungodly" embellishments of the greatest artists of the day.

The storm clouds, which had threatened before we left the little chapel, opened with sudden fury as we reached the San Pietro gate. Dampened, we found shelter of a kind under its archway. The outburst was the first of the autumn and, consequently, of more than a little intensity. Knowing Fiammetta's purpose in Assisi, I wondered whether the wind and the rain were a signal of St Francis's displeasure or merely

---

* The Porziuncola is the little chapel that witnessed the birth of the Franciscan order. Close by is the cell, or infirmary, where St Francis died. Today, both are incorporated within the basilica of Santa Maria degli Angeli. – J.G.
** Paul Baldassare is here referring to the Roman league, about two and one third English miles. – J.G.

an indication that in death he had become resigned to man's follies and was welcoming us by bringing a freshness to the air and rinsing the alleys of their filth.

"When I was a child," Fiammetta began. I held her close to protect her from the spray driven beneath the arch. "When I was a child," she repeated with emphasis, aware that my mind was more occupied with her body than her words, "my father brought many artists of talent under his patronage. My favourite was one as ill-favoured as his paintings were beautiful. Giotto was kind to me; he made me laugh and, had his artistic genius deserted him, his ready wit would have secured him a place as my father's jester. I loved him with a child's adoration; when he left us, I wept for days." There was an undeniable catch in her voice as she spoke of him.

"Even before his death, it was said he had transformed the art of painting. Now we shall see how true that is!"

As swiftly as it had begun, the rain ceased, remembered only by the vapour lazily rising from the cobbles and rooftops. The sun, blazing from a newly-washed sky, accompanied us to the doors of the church. For some moments we stood silently within the lower basilica waiting for our sight to return. Gradually the form of the building took shape until at last I was able to see its decorations emerge from the gloom in all their exquisite beauty. I had quite expected Fiammetta to take me first to the paintings of her favourite but instead she played on my emotions, leading me to the right transept and Cimabue's Madonna with its sad St Francis at Her side. When I had admired this to her satisfaction she walked me slowly round the paintings of Martini and the two Lorenzini brothers, drawing my attention in particular to Martini's much stronger depiction of the Saint. When next she stopped, it was before scenes of the Nativity and life of Christ. Unable to control her sobbing, she clung to me.

"These are by my old friend," she managed to say. "Are they not truly wonderful?"

Indeed they were. By comparison, the paintings we had already seen were flat and lifeless though, if I could trust my artistic sense, the work of Cimabue had been a brave attempt to break with tradition. Giotto had succeeded where his master had failed. His figures were so imbued with life I could almost feel their breath upon my face.

"There are more." Fiammetta, tears still in her eyes, led the way to the upper basilica. Here, in frescos of unbelievable spiritual power and movement, Giotto had recreated the life of St Francis within a world of delightful simplicity. In these paintings he had surpassed the Giotto of the lower basilica: never before had life been expressed with such truthfulness and sensitivity.

For many days we returned to the church, lost in wonder at both painter and subjects. On our last visit Fiammetta was in a strange, other-worldly mood.

"These paintings of Giotto's will have a greater influence on your life, dear Paul, than you can possibly imagine. They will prove to be one of the means whereby you are drawn closer to your goal." She turned towards me with a look that penetrated my innermost being. She seemed not to be herself – and then, intuitively, I knew Telesphorus was speaking through her. But what was he telling me? Belabour my mind though I would, it was beyond my understanding. How could an artist influence medicine. I might ask the question now; the answer lay in the future.

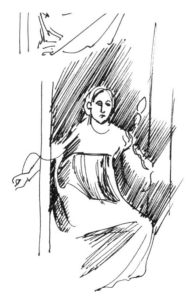

Never before had life been expressed with such truthfulness and sensitivity. Detail of Girl carding wool by Giotto (Arena Chapel, Padua).

Before the winds of winter came we returned to Naples by roads still easily passable. Our villa, a mile or two outside the city, had been given to Fiammetta by her father and here we rested from our travels. In the early hours of the day we had breakfast brought to us on the gallery around the inner courtyard. We occupied ourselves by reading, shaded from the rising sun by the foliage of a profusion of climbing plants. The flowers below sweetened the air with the freshness of their perfume. On days when we chose not to seek entertainment in the city, we would spend our afternoons in the walled garden, the beauty of which reminded me of a corner of my estate in Constantinople. Around and across the garden were walks covered with trellises of vines and walled in by roses and jasmine. In the middle a lawn of lushest green was planted with patterned flower borders, ornamental trees and flowering shrubs – the scent of their blooms in their seasons brought joy to the senses. In its very centre lay a carved white marble basin from which arose a fountain in the form of two intertwined lovers. The water sprang high in the air, tumbling back with music in its fall into the basin from where it was taken through hidden channels to refresh the garden. Days spent with Fiammetta in that heaven on earth were enchantment indeed.

Strolling together hand-in-hand in the balm of a summer twilight, making our way to the readied bower where we would sleep, all passion spent, I said something that I must have said in different ways almost every day.

"This garden is blest," I murmured. "Whatever the season, whatever the weather; in rain, wind, or sun it shows a different aspect. But it is always beautiful; it never ceases to please and delight. It was created for our love!"

Her response surprised me. Instead of squeezing my hand in silent agreement and drawing closer to me, she said simply and in a matter of fact tone:

"There are flies, even in Paradise."

Although I banished from my mind the unwelcome sense of foreboding that this conjured up, her words returned to haunt me before another year was passed.

It was spring again. Each year at about this time I returned to Salerno. Despite my misgiving at the direction orthodox medicine seemed to be taking – if, indeed, it had not already entered a dead-end – I was resolved to keep a watchful eye on its travails. I was away for three weeks.

On my return I could not escape the fearful disaster that had overtaken the land. Terror crowded the streets of Naples and when I arrived home, it was to find the servants fled save for Fiammetta's young handmaid whose bare arms were disfigured by ugly livid blotches. Bidding me not to touch her, she hurried ahead to Fiammetta's bedroom.

"Yes, my beloved, there *are* flies in Paradise! Come, let me hold you that we may leave this world together."

I fell to my knees at the bedside and took her in my arms.

With her dying breath, Fiammetta kissed me.

*   *   *

Fiammetta had been Boccaccio's inspiration, both in his life and in his work. I knew, from reports received from Florence, that he loved her still and continued to live in the belief that one day she would tire of her current lover and return to him. Since it was eminently possible, given the present state of the country, that word of her death would never reach him, I resolved to travel to Florence with the news that Fiammetta was lost to both of us for ever – though I would spare him the knowledge that Fiammetta/Ishtar could never have been his.

I gathered a bodyguard of the soundest fighting men left in Naples and ensured their loyalty: money is the answer to many things. We carried our needs with us and rode across country by uncommon tracks. At night we made camp in the open and far from human habitation. I strictly forbade the men to come close to other people.

The journey was one of unmitigated horror. Even in the remotest regions we encountered citizens who had fled their homes, their possessions, and their families in the hope that God would not pursue them with His wrath but intended to destroy only those who remained within the city walls. Their mistaken belief was everywhere in evidence in the foul pollution that assailed the senses.

Free from the pestilence, we were admitted to Florence. My enquiries, however, elicited the fact that Boccaccio was living at Corbignano. Much to my relief, and with all possible speed, we abandoned the city.

The Boccaccio I found at Corbignano was the not the Boccaccio who had left Naples seven years previously. A deep melancholy had settled on him and when he learnt of Fiammetta's death he shut himself in his room and wept unceasingly for three days. When he emerged he had purged himself of his grief and, knowing now that Fiammetta was truly beyond his recall, he seemed to have prepared himself to face reality once again.

Although we had little in common he urged me to stay. He wished to talk, not only about Fiammetta – he felt he had seven lost years to regain and showed no jealousy when I recounted their joys and delights. I, too, was happy to hear him speak about the Fiammetta I had never known. Our talk released my numbed emotions and I was able to view the world, not with an uncomprehending vision, but as it was – and it was worse, far worse, than I had feared.

Boccaccio was insistent on describing for me the ravages of the pestilence now sweeping with devastating fury throughout Europe. It was as if he was driven to rehearse a story he was intending to use in another place.* His tale, indeed, left nothing to my imagination.

The deadly pestilence had, he said, originated some years earlier in the East from where it had pursued its relentless progress into the West, consuming uncountable lives along the way. Whether it had been brought upon mankind by the influence of celestial bodies or had been sent by God in His just wrath as punishment for their sins was of little consequence in the presence of its mighty destructive power.

"We took every precaution that came to mind to prevent the disease from entering Florence." Boccaccio spoke as lucidly as he wrote. "We appointed officials to clean the city and we refused entry to all who were sick. Those who believed the pestilence to be a visitation from God, addressed their humble supplications to Him in the churches and in processions through the city. But it was all to no avail and in the spring the pestilence breached the city's defences in all its horror."

What, I asked, were its manifestations, for all I had seen had been its awesome consequences.

"They are not as they were in the East, where a sudden bleeding

---

* Dr Baldassare's instinct was correct. Boccaccio's account of the Black Death in Florence appears in the introductory paragraphs of the stories of the first day of the *Decameron*. It is perhaps of interest that in his written description Boccaccio states that the pestilence (bubonic plague) raged from March to July. The flea that spreads the disease does so through its bite, but only when the plague bacilli form a blockage with fibrinous matter in its gut. A blocked flea makes repeated attempts to feed on blood, but since it cannot get the blood to pass the blockage, it regurgitates masses of plague bacilli into the bite wound. Curiously, the blockage clears at temperatures above 80°F; consequently epidemics of plague subside spontaneously when the ambient temperature exceeds this level. – J.G.

from the nose was a sure sign of impending death*. In European countries, in men and women alike, swellings appear in the groin or armpits – these are about the size of an egg or an apple; some larger, some smaller; the people call them gavoccioli**. They soon spread indiscriminately to all parts of the body. After a while the illness begins to change form with the appearance of black spots or livid marks, often on the arm or thigh, some few and large, some minute and numerous. Both swellings and spots are invariable tokens of approaching death."

He stopped abruptly and for a minute or two sat gazing inwardly. Fiammetta was in his thoughts as she was in mine. Pouring some wine, he waved a request that I did the same. "And how do the physicians treat the disease?" I enquired. He gave a start, almost spilling the wine, gathered his thoughts and continued.

"Nothing influences the disease, neither the art of the physician nor the virtues of physic. Whether it is in the nature of the illness to defy treatment or whether the physicians are at fault, being in ignorance of its source and thus failing to apply the correct remedy, I know not. Besides, many, both men and women practise without the least knowledge of medicine. Few recover and many of those who die, do so within three days of the appearance of their symptoms and in most cases without fever or any other manifestation!

"The pestilence is deadly beyond belief. It is conveyed from the sick to the healthy merely by speech or association. Its virulence is such that should a healthy person touch the clothes of the sick or anything that has been used by them, they seem to contract the disease. The energy of the contagion is startling.

"Those who remain alive," he said, "shun, each in their own way, all contact with the sick and their belongings. Some think that to live temperately and avoid all excess is the best means of preserving their health. They have banded together and formed communities in houses free of the sickness. Others take their pleasure in song and merriment, indulging the satisfaction of every appetite.

"Between these two," Boccaccio continued – I was as fascinated by this tale of human misery as if by a cobra poised to strike – "are those who keep to a middle course. They walk abroad carrying flowers or

---

* The pneumonic form of plague. – J.G.
** Buboes. – J.G.

fragrant herbs or spices which they frequently raise to their noses, believing it an excellent thing to give comfort to their brains with such perfumes as an antidote to the stench emitted by the dead and dying. But whatever the course of action adopted, many die.

"The world is changing, my friend. Life will never be the same again." Boccaccio's voice was hesitant with emotion. His happiness had been destroyed and now that Fiammetta was dead he was deprived even of hope. But it was not his personal world he was mourning; it was the life of all mankind on this earth.

"In consequence of the dearth of servants and the neglect of the sick, the previously unthinkable is happening," he continued his story. "No woman, however fastidious, fair or well-born she may be, shrinks, when sick, from the ministrations of a man whether young or old. She does not scruple to expose to him every part of her body with no more shame than if he were a woman, and submits to whatever necessity her disease demands. This has resulted, among those who recover, in a loss of modesty. Citizens who have heard of this – let alone those who have witnessed its occurrence – are struck dumb with amazement. The effect, which is not to be wondered at with death ever present night and day, is that practices contrary to their former conduct have taken root among the survivors.

"How many families of historic fame, of vast ancestral lands, of proverbial wealth, now have none to continue the succession!" A note of despairing sadness entered his voice. "How many brave men, how many fair ladies, how many gallant youths, whom any physician, were he Galen, Hippocrates or Aesculapius himself, would have pronounced in the soundest of health, breakfasted with their kinsfolk, comrades and friends in the morning and, when the evening came, supped with their forefathers in the next world!"

Boccaccio sank back in his chair, exhausted from the emotions aroused by the telling of the tale, and entered his own other world of lost love and creative fantasy. He spoke not another word in my presence.

12

An alchemist sees what he has convinced himself he will see*

Boccaccio *was* right. The world *would* never be the same again. By the time the pestilence had run its course that terrible summer, upward of one hundred thousand citizens of Florence were supping with their forefathers. Many had lain putrefying in the streets before their mortal bodies had been thrown with less ceremony than would have been accorded a goat, into a common trench. At every church, pits were dug down to the water level and the poor who had died in the night were bundled up and thrown in. The next morning, earth was shovelled over them; later others were cast on top with another layer of earth, just as one would make lasagne with layers of pasta and cheese**. For three more years the plague flowed and ebbed throughout Europe with the same mournful consequences, sparing no city, no countryside. And that was just the beginning.

Death was the ever-present spectre. A second Flood was confidently predicted. Comets and meteors were interpreted as signs of God's wrath. Every event that seemed to contradict nature was a call to mankind to repent and atone for his sins. And God did not stop at warning; He punished. He constantly sent new epidemics of plague, both bubonic and pneumonic, to destroy the cities and lay waste the land. The

---

* Alchemy and the belief in the philosophers' stone and in the Fountain of Youth. 1348–1516. – J.G.
** Dr Baldassare has borrowed this metaphor from Boccaccio. – J.G.

unknown took a hand in the shape of new, terrifying, diseases. People were taken with the English sweat and other strange fevers. The dancing mania added to the horror as those caught in its grip defied their fate to the last moment as they sank exhausted into death. [One form of this mania, Dr Annandale, may have been due to the use of grain, especially rye, contaminated with the ergot fungus. Inevitably, it led to waves of hysterical imitation. The English sweat remains unidentified, though it may have been influenza.]

And there was famine. Starving, panic-stricken peasants abandoned their homes, compelled by some incomprehensible drive to wander, to escape to a better land. Unable to find it, they formed themselves into marauding bands to plunder and ravage wherever the spirit took them, until eventually their excesses were put down with a cruelty that surpassed their own.

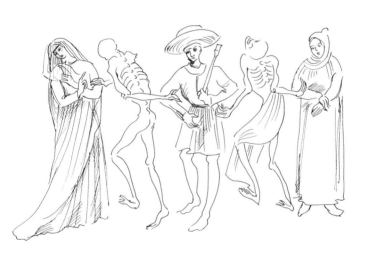

One of the frescos of the Dance of Death in the Church of La Chaise-Dieu showing, from the left, the noble lady, the knight and the young lady.

The fear of death permeated every aspect of life, not as an intellectual curiosity about the hereafter, but as a real, morbid state of mind. Christianity may have preached the defeat of Death, in the sense of death being the gateway to a new (and better) life, but it could not conquer the fear of extinction which took outward shape in a powerful imagery. Death was seen as the reaper with his sickle, the hunter with his bow and arrow, and, in company with War, Rebellion and Famine, as one of the four horsemen of the Apocalypse. The unrepentant newly dead were accompanied by Death, the piper, in a ghastly dance across the graves and burial pits from which arose the decomposed corpses still wearing the clothes appropriate to their estate. The dead were robbed of the peace promised them in the requiem mass.

Whenever an epidemic of plague or pestilence was feared or entered a parish, this dance of Death was painted on the walls of churches* and cemeteries – not just as a warning call to repentance, decency and morality, but also in the hope of foiling the power of Death through his image.

Yet, distant and objective observer though I was of a society in decay, as the years passed I detected a more subtle upheaval. In memory's eye, I was back with Giotto's frescos in Assisi seeing again art announcing change, but with a greater certainty. No longer was the message conveyed by the dance contained in a pictorial sermon. Instead, the artists allowed their pictures to speak for themselves by showing how Death surprised man in the midst of life**. "Death," these pictures said, "may come with violence and destruction or be welcomed as friend and liberator; man himself, by the way he shapes his life, makes the choice." They were plainly indicating that in the intellectual movement*** now in progress, Christian man was displacing his God by planting himself firmly at the centre of the world – and, in so doing, lessening his confrontation with matters not of this sphere.

The scientific discoveries of the time seemed only to make matters worse. The hidden was being illuminated but, by contrast, the only mystery that really concerned the people – the mystery of existence – was being plunged ever deeper into darkness. And their superstitious natures were being fanned by the visions of St John the Divine recorded in the Book of Revelations and thundered abroad by every vagabond prophet who could read. I could make little sense of this apparent paradox: religious and social confusion on the one hand, and a freeing of the intellect to permit a cultural flowering on the other.

---

* A fine example is still to be seen in the Church of La Chaise-Dieu, Haute Loire. – J.G.
** For instance, Hans Holbein's pictures in *Les Simulachres et Histoirees Faces de la Mort*. – J.G.
*** The Renaissance. – J.G.

I travelled the length and breadth of Italy in search of an answer; on the purely material plane this could be found in the economic, social and political conditions that now prevailed in the north of Italy. Yet this was not the entire story; there was something more and that something was analogous to the wisdom that comes with the years as the body grows old. And the most noticeable change was in the people's outlook on life. I experienced it also north of the Alps, modified only insofar as the humours of these peoples differed from those of their more sensual southern neighbours. I even wondered whether I, too, was experiencing this same change in my state of mind.

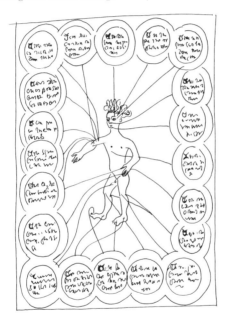

Should the sick call on the services of a physician he might well decide that the best remedy was the letting of blood. This chart, dating from the end of the fourteenth century, indicates the most suitable site for the letting of blood as determined by the patient's symptoms.

Medicine was, at first, unaffected by the intellectual upheaval – though I knew in the end escape would be impossible. But until this time came, the sick continued to rely on what worked for them – whether this required the services of a herbalist, a uroscopist, an astrologer, a magician, an apothecary, an alchemist or a physician. If the affliction was one of exquisite pain and the patient knew its cause, he might call upon a drawer of teeth, a cutter for stone or a coucher for cataract. But the most fortunate were those blessed with a woman of the house who could draw upon the experience of her mother and her mother before her.

Since the followers of traditional humoral and Galenic teachings were stumbling along in a trackless desert, I decided to take a closer look at alchemy. As always, when the main road fails, man takes to alternative pathways.

*   *   *

The next morning I awoke to find Telesphorus standing at my bedhead.

"Yes, Master, I know what is in your mind and I have returned to see that you come to no harm. Although Gerber gave the material aspects of alchemy a semblance of respectability some seven centuries ago, its well-nigh impenetrable symbolism hides many secrets that may, to the uninitiated, be spiritually harmful. You may think that my return implies a measure of approval of your action, but you would be wrong – as I shall show you. You, Paul Balthasar, are pursuing alchemy believing the discovery of the philosophers' stone is the route to both wealth and a medicine to cure all mankind's ills – a panacea, in fact. But remember my father's words: Panacea will always be sought by man, but she will be forever inaccessible.

"I, however, know that in one of its many aspects, alchemy will overturn the past and open a new sphere of medical knowledge – if not of understanding. You must appreciate that alchemy is a turbulent conglomeration of matters chemical, mystical, and theological with its roots grasping through undercurrents of astrology and magic. So, I must acquaint you with its past. For, if a man had only the experience of his own lifetime to call upon, his knowledge would be commensurate with the shortness of his existence."

Telesphorus beamed at me, his eyes twinkling with delight. "I learnt that at school on Mount Olympus!" It was a long while since I had seen him so pleased with himself.

"But for now, let us eat and prepare ourselves for the day. Then I shall walk with you through the woods and meadows and take you back to school."

*   *   *

"Whatever view you take of alchemy, it is submerged in symbolism," was Telesphorus's not very encouraging start. It also warned me that he was about to deliver a lecture in truly magisterial manner.

"Although al-kimia is the Arabic origin of the name, alchemy extends back through Greece to Egypt." By his tone I knew I was correct about his intentions. "In its purest form it was concerned with the transmutation of the lower nature into the higher or Divine nature; it represented man's desire to achieve union with God. But this very soon became inextricably entangled with his baser struggle to wrest from Nature her most closely guarded secrets. The ancient Chaldeans believed that there were spirits in all things and that these could be extracted by fire. They named the spirits according to their origin: collectively they were regarded as the soul of the world – the source of life. This is why, Balthasar, their furnaces are so important to the alchemists of today.

"Astrology was next to complicate the issue by postulating that the seven planets – the sun, moon, Mars, Mercury, Jupiter, Saturn and Venus – corresponded to the seven days of the week and to the seven metals – gold, silver, iron, quicksilver, tin, lead and copper. These metals were all believed to be, in essence, the same as one another and to be generated in the very bowels of the earth. Here they ripened into gold, the purest and noblest of them all. The alchemists deceived themselves into thinking they could speed the process.

"They considered mercury to be the closest to gold, lacking only a certain something to give it the required colour and solidity. The missing something was thought to be related to sulphur and, indeed, the Arabic name for the philosophers' stone – al-kibrit al-ahmar – may be translated as red sulphur.

"Through some rather tortuous thinking, they next decided that by transmuting base metals into gold they could also discover an elixir of life, a cure for all ills and the guarantor of immortality. They called this their aurum potabile, their golden cordial."

I hid my face in my hands and sighed at the folly of mankind.

"Ah! I see the possibility of eternal youth for everyman fills you with pity – or is it horror?" Telesphorus was genuine in his sympathy. "But let me reassure you. It will never come to pass. I shall explain in a moment. First, I must delve a little deeper into the symbolism of alchemy.

"The central symbol is the marriage of sulphur and quicksilver – the metal, mercury – which are also the sun and the moon, the king and the queen. This is important because, since his Fall, man has been divided and spiritually weakened. He can only become his true spiritual self again once the two forces that split him apart have become reconciled. So – and here, Balthasar, you may see an analogy with your own predicament – that reconciliation is expressed alchemically through the union of male and female – the marriage of the soul's male and female entities: the images of the Spirit and the soul.

"However – and there is always a catch, is there not? – the king and the queen may be killed at the moment of their wedding and, buried together, rise up in rejuvenated union.

"Now, Paul Balthasar, I shall express what I have said in terms that are relevant to you and so may be more readily comprehensible.

"A man is not a complete person; neither is a woman. At the beginning of time when the gods put life upon the earth, they divided the essential life force of each being into two parts. At first, these parts – man and woman – were undifferentiated, so the gods decided to clothe them differently before throwing them into the maelstrom of life*. Not every being is re-united here, which is why the realization of love is often impossible. Many human beings have to grasp at what they imagine to be love when, in fact, it is only a mirage – an illusion.

"Balthasar, a man is not wholly man, in him is more or less of woman. A woman is not wholly woman, in her is more or less of man. This may explain the behaviour of some you meet, particularly in their relationships one with another. The body may be that of a man, yet the spirit that of a woman. The two parts may be equally blended to give woman now, man tomorrow."

By now our walk had returned us to my home and as we entered, Telesphorus, ever sensitive to my wishes, led me to my room. Gradually my ears closed to his words and his voice grew more and more distant. My world became silent.

I had fallen asleep. My mind could absorb no more.

I awoke as dawn was breaking. I never cease to marvel at the beauty Nature can unfold when she chooses. I watched, spellbound, as her colours deftly changed in hue and brightness as night's lingering clouds

* Telesphorus had evidently been reading Plato's *Symposium*! – J.G.

caught the rays of the rising sun and sped them back to earth. When next I looked, all was gone and there in a sky, the blue of Ishtar's eyes, the sun reigned supreme.

Turning from the window, I saw that Telesphorus had entered the room and been watching the miracle as entranced as I.

"Good morning, Master," he said softly. "I sense your mood is well suited to the story I shall tell today.

"You know," he continued, "that one of the prizes sought by world-blinded alchemists is not to be won: Panacea will never return. Their quest for the elixir of life, for the immortality to allow them to enjoy to the full the fruits of their labours, also is doomed to everlasting failure."

As the sun climbed towards its zenith, we began our walk in the welcome shade of the woods. At each step the scent of plants trodden, unavoidably, under foot rose to please our senses.

"But, Balthasar," he adopted once again his magisterial tone, "nothing, it seems, can awaken your race from its dream of perpetual youth enriched with the knowledge of maturity!" And he proceeded to pour out a deplorably long list of instances of mankind's credulity. My attention returned when he arrived at his last, and most recent, example.

"... And then, a year or two after he had taken Puerto Rico, Juan Ponce de Léon mounted an expedition to find the Fountain of Youth in the New World. He was mightily upset at failing to do so." [What, Dr Annandale, he discovered instead was Florida! The amusing irony of this will not, I am sure, be lost on you. His expedition nonetheless demonstrated the influence exerted by the legend of the fountain on the practical affairs of those days. The search for perpetual youth – or, at least, for rejuvenation – still continues in your day with people throwing their money away on the likes of specific sera, monkey glands, transplantation of human testicles and various imaginative potions and injections.]

The lesson concluded, we completed our walk in comparative silence, rejoicing in small things: the wild cyclamen nestling in clumps between the rocks, our feet idly kicking fir cones along the path. I was as close to happiness as I could come without Ishtar at my side. Fortunately Telesphorus was too absorbed in his own thoughts to read mine, but even if he had he would have seen he was part of my present contentment – a state that was not to last much longer.

"Tomorrow," he announced, as we bade each other goodnight,

"tomorrow I shall take you to the laboratory of Johannes Tritheim where you shall witness a marvel more magnificent than the transmutation of base metal into gold: the creation of life itself!" And before I could gather myself, he had disappeared into his room and closed the door. I heard the bolt pushed to.

We opened the heavy oak door to Trithemius's dungeon-like cell to be assaulted by a fearsome stench compared to which the reek of putrid flesh was as the odour of sweet violets. Feeling our way down the treacherous steps we saw its source. Bent over his furnace, a filthy leather apron wrapped around his waist, the alchemist was pumping away with his bellows at the flames beneath a steaming iron cauldron. Constantly glancing up at an hour-glass, suspended from a long iron peg driven into the overhanging chimney breast, he ensured the safe passage of every grain of sand. Behind him, his long clay pipe rested on a three-legged stool. The only light seemed to come from the furnace itself – the windows were encrusted with grime and what little light did penetrate was obstructed by piles of books filling the deep embrasures. All around were littered the instruments and symbols of his calling.

Trithemius ignored us until the last grain of sand had fallen through. Then he coughed, a deep bubbling cough rising from the very bases of his lungs, and turned his bloodshot eyes towards us. He gave no greeting and we responded in like fashion.

"Man's struggle to create life has been recorded in myth and legend." The intensity of the sound emerging from the alchemist's plump round body was spellbinding. "He has attempted to awaken the dead and to make new life to spring from the decay of corpses. It is said that many centuries ago a Jew created stags from cucumbers and roebuck from gourds*. But no one has created life in human form." Trithemius paused and peered into the stinking cauldron. "Until now!

"Within this cauldron," his voice reverberated within the stone walls, "there lies a work of God, a miracle; the food to nourish the human life I shall create. It is the arcana sanguinis humani**. It is the food that has eluded all my predecessors."

---

* In the first century AD by Jehoshua ben Hamanjah with the aid of the book of Jeziriah – according to the Jerusalem Talmud. – J.G.
** Being "a work of God", the nature of the arcana sanguinis humani is destined to remain mysterious and a secret until the end of time. – J.G.

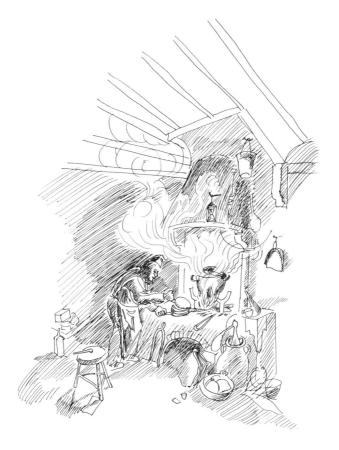

We opened the heavy oak door to Trithemius's dungeon-like cell... Bent over his furnace, a filthy leather apron wrapped around his waist, the alchemist was pumping away with his bellows at the flames beneath a steaming iron cauldron.

At this point Trithemius acknowledged our presence, not out of courtesy but because he wished the recognition of his genius. Like two obedient children we uttered a few appropriate words in Latin which seemed to give him pleasure.

"Hitherto they, myself included, have implanted human semen into a member of the cucumber family putrefying in the natural heat of horse dung. After forty days in a glass retort, the material begins to stir and to take the shape of a transparent embryo. No man has progressed beyond this, because no man has possessed the food of further life. Now, I have it at my disposal!" Trithemius was exultant.

He said nothing more until the sand had once again run through the glass. He stood, unmoving, gazing at the cauldron.

"You have no children?" He raised his head and spoke directly and curtly at me.

"No," I answered, "although I have known many women."

"Then you are of no use. Why did you come? Your assistant," indicating Telesphorus, "had said you wished to assist me in my greatest experiment."

Telesphorus had once again taken a hand in determining the course of my life.

"Trithemius, I cannot have made my meaning plain." Telesphorus, ever the tactful soother of irate emotions, spoke for the first time. "I had hoped you might allow my Master to observe this greatest of all alchemical experiments and to encourage and reinforce the spiritual power you will conjure up."

"Tonight I am host to two couples who have undertaken to obey my instructions and to lie together as the dawn begins to break." Trithemius was mollified and eager for my "spiritual" help. "When the sounds of their coupling have ceased you, my renowned physician, shall collect the material I require – though when your assistant told me of your great talents I had intended to dismiss one of the men and use you as a giver of seed. Evidently, your seed lacks sufficient life force." He was not an expert in veiling his insults.

Nevertheless, I agreed to do as he wished and the next morning I visited the two bedrooms and removed the semen from inside the women. I took both portions to the adjoining chapel where Trithemius awaited. He was standing by a table at the chancel steps bathed in the early morning light. On the table were two glass retorts, the sides of which were translucent, with the vapours rising from the ugly glutinous masses at their bottoms.

Trithemius took the semen from me and introduced one portion into each retort.

"My method of gathering the semen is unique." His voice was hushed; even he was overawed by his surroundings and the enormity of what he was attempting. "Moreover, I have added a human afterbirth to the dung to create the most natural conditions for success – and success is ensured by the perfection of the astrological aspects at this moment. It will be many years before all the conjunctions are again favourable."

During our stay, we were treated in a more civilized manner than I had expected. Trithemius's house was comfortably furnished and we were well attended by his servants. He himself sometimes appeared at table looking clean and presentable in his clerical garb, but mostly he occupied his days in the sordid surroundings of his laboratory where he was pleased that I should watch and, sometimes, help.

Toward the end of the forty days of waiting – during which time we neither of us entered the chapel – he grew agitated. This increased until, unable to concentrate on his work, he confided in me.

"As a man of God, I am disturbed by the consequences should I succeed. I am thinking of Maimonides, the only man to have created a homunculus. Although his experiment was re-creation and not creation, my dilemma is the same as his.

"With the promise that he would bring him back to life and with his agreement, Maimonides cut up the living body of his pupil, Menasse. The pieces, he sprinkled with the perfume of the 'plant of life', the 'balsam of immortality' and an extract of the 'flower of the strength of life' and let them lie under a glass vessel. On the fourth day he saw that the tissues had begun to melt and to rearrange themselves.

"After five months he could recognize the human form; after six months nerves and blood vessels became apparent; and in the seventh month he saw the first movements. Then, he realized the catastrophe that would result as soon as people saw the revitalized corpse: they would worship him and thereby lose their reverence for God. In the eighth month Menasse smiled at him.

"In utter desperation, Maimonides weighed his promise to bring his pupil back to life against his duty to preserve humanity from incalculable disaster. He laid his conflict before a meeting of wise men who decided that, for the honour of God, Maimonides must break his oath and take the life of a being created under such unusual circumstances. This he did.

"Balthasar, do *I* continue?" Trithemius was in mental agony, but my curiosity outweighed my sense.

"Trithemius," I said, "you shall pursue the experiment to its conclusion. Should it succeed, *then* let us face the consequences."

[Observe, Dr Annandale, how I reacted like one of your "pure" scientists searching for his Holy Grail with no thought of a practical application and a total disregard of the consequences should he be successful.]

"I have two days until I must begin feeding my creations." He looked searchingly into my face, as if seeking irresolution on my part. "You, Balthasar, have given me the strength to carry my work to its conclusion. I shall pray for us both. May God have mercy on us!"

The two days passed and at dawn on the third we entered the chapel. Life was stirring in both retorts; it was of a pale colour in one and of a darker in the other. Trithemius carefully introduced a small quantity of arcana sanguinis humani into each retort reading, as he did so, a long incantation from a book produced from under his apron. For forty more days he repeated the ritual, and each day we watched the life assume increasingly recognizable human shape.

On the forty-first day, a thunderstorm [obligatory, are they not, Dr Annandale, in situations of this nature?] was raging as we approached the chancel, lightning filled the chapel and the two retorts shattered. There was no noise apart from the instantaneous clap of thunder; gently the glass sides fell away to the table top, leaving two perfectly formed human figures standing in their places. Both were female, of the height that would be expected of a new-born, but both were unmistakably fully mature adults in miniature. One was fair skinned; one was dark.

Trithemius gazed at his creations in silence, unable to believe what he had done. Then, as the significance of it penetrated his mind, he fell to his knees and began to whimper. It was the sound of man suddenly made mad.

I, too, was gazing at the figures, but in greater horror than Trithemius can ever have felt. I knew who he had created. Ishtar and Allatu! For the next hour, I stood transfixed as they slowly grew to adult size. The first to speak was Ishtar.

"Bal-sarra-uzur, you have committed a mortal sin. It is given only to the gods to create life."

Before she could say more, Allatu took her by the hand as she had done all those centuries ago. With the force at Allatu's command passing into her, Ishtar began to lose shape and, with sickening slowness, to dissolve into slime.

My screaming joined with Trithemius's whimpering in a requiem that must have been born in hell for there could be no hope of eternal rest for any in that chapel on that day. And all the while we were subjected to the contempt of Allatu, glorying in her power and naked sensuousness.

"Yes, Bal-sarra-uzur, you have indeed sinned, and madness shall not save you from the knowledge of that sin." The look she gave Trithemius was almost one of pity. "Man cannot meddle in the work of the gods and escape unscathed!" With which she leaned forward and touched Trithemius over his heart. His whimpering ceased as he slumped to the ground.

"And you, Bal-sarra-uzur, you I leave once more to weep for Ishtar." And she was gone.

*   *   *

The fire had started from Trithemius's untended furnace and spread throughout the buildings despite the desperate efforts of the servants and the rain which lashed down furiously all day. The chapel was completely burnt out; only a shell remained and everything within it was destroyed beyond recognition.

Telesphorus had rescued me before the fire had taken a hold.

"Bal-sarra-uzur, what you experienced with Trithemius was only an illusion. Man is a strange and susceptible creature. When his convictions are strong enough, what he wants – what he expects – to see, he *will* see." Was I imagining it or did I really hear him say, "Maybe, though, your illusion will be a future reality"?

[The extension of the concept of the homunculus, Dr Annandale, into modern times (for instance, in-vitro fertilization, cloning, the freezing of embryos and similar practices) is the ultimate achievement of the Renaissance and entirely negates all spiritual values surrounding the mystery of life. Man has now well and truly displaced God from the centre of the universe. Does it also prove there is no God?]

13

*Anatomy steps out of the mediaeval shadows**

or a while during his adolescent years, Paracelsus had been apprenticed to Trithemius. Subsequently he, too, made use of arcana sanguinis humani in his attempts to create a homunculus, not in the least deterred by his old master's fate. If Paracelsus is to be believed – and there is, admittedly, little reason to do so – his father, a respectable, educated physician, taught him medicine, botany, natural philosophy, and mineralogy and mining. The fact that the first determined his choice of career and the last the direction it would take, is evidence only of the atmosphere in which he was raised and not of the reality of an education.

In our wanderings throughout Europe the paths of Paracelsus and myself never crossed. If they had, I doubt that we would have suited each other, for he was a braggart and arrogant to the point of insanity, preaching the unintelligible with an astounding degree of incoherence. Nevertheless, he acquired a considerable number of eminent (and intelligent) men as his patients. Although I knew of his reputation during his lifetime, it was not until a year or so after his death that I learned of his spectacular influence on the course of medicine.

At a time when the printing houses of Europe were vying with one another over the quality of their typography, that of Herbst in Basle excelled thanks to the work of Joannes Oporinus. This man was no

*Paracelsus, art and printing break the shackles of mediaeval medicine. Second quarter of the 16th century. – J.G.

160

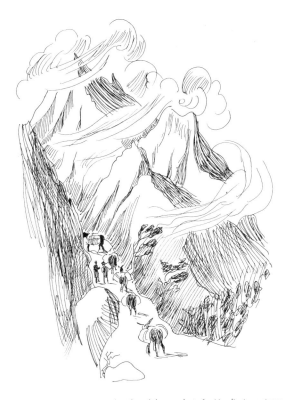

Oporinus oversees the transport across the Alps of the woodcuts for Vesalius's anatomy strapped to the sides of mules.

ordinary printer for he was professor of Greek at the University and had, on occasion, been Paracelsus's amanuensis. His reputation was such that when Vesalius was seeking a printer for his monumental text on anatomy, he chose Oporinus. There was, however, a problem: the woodcuts were in Padua and the printing house was on the other side of the Alps in Basle. The difficulty was resolved by Oporinus's agreeing to oversee their transport strapped to the sides of mules. As I had already been in Padua for some years while Vesalius dissected and Jan Calcar prepared his exquisite illustrations, I took the opportunity to move on. [I would, Dr Annandale, have described Calcar's illustrations as incomparable but that would not have been strictly true. The anatomical drawings made by Leonardo da Vinci in his notebooks between fifty and sixty years earlier are artistically superior. Although Galenic elements appear in the earlier of these, the later ones are more detailed and realistic and are accompanied by extensive notes. Regrettably, Leonardo drew for himself and did not publish (although a planned Galenic anatomic atlas never came to fruition) and his notebooks inexplicably disappeared from view until the end of the nineteenth century.]

Knowing the cargo of our little caravan to be beyond price, we were in a state of almost constant agitation lest one of the animals should lose its footing among the clouds and disappear over a precipice; but I believe we were in the greater danger of that hazard ourselves. Since all I know about Paracelsus I learnt from Oporinus, I shall record the story as he related it to me during that treacherous journey:

* * *

Paracelsus (Oporinus began), Paracelsus – I shall call him that, even though he did not assume the name until some years later – left Trithemius with his head full of an avalanche of magic, mysticism and chemistry. His obsession with the alchemical belief that the seven metals were generated in the bowels of the earth led him to the mining school run by the Fuggers at Huttenberg and then to Sigismund Fueger's mine at Schwaz, where he investigated the chemical properties of various metallic substances*.

The urge to be a physician had already taken hold of him and his reticence about where he had studied made me suspect that at the start he had simply relied on the knowledge gained from being his father's son and from his astute observation of the world around him. He was constantly on the move, never staying in one place for long because, as he said, "A physician must be a traveller, since he must enquire of the world." And enquire he most certainly did, not of authority but of the people – for preference gypsies, keepers of bath houses, fortune tellers, executioners and his drinking companions in the more disreputable taverns. In this manner he acquired considerable expertise in folk-medicine and a good grasp of what would succeed and what

---

* The Fuggers were an extremely wealthy family of German merchants founded in the fourteenth century by Johann Fugger. As was not unusual, the name was variously spelt. Paracelsus also left a meticulously observed account of the diseases prevalent among the miners. This could be regarded as the first work on occupational diseases and was probably the only rational thing he wrote. – J.G.

would fail. Frequently, those he attended were cured when other physicians had despaired.

His contempt for authority, both past and present, was formidable and he had the temerity to write and lecture in German, not in Latin – something no one aspiring to even a modicum of learning would contemplate. Through the good offices of Erasmus, one of his distinguished patients, he was appointed physician to the city of Basle, a position carrying with it the responsibility of lecturing to the medical faculty. On the first occasion he was, as usual when lecturing, half-drunk – the complete state he reserved for his visits to the sick – and began, I remember, by announcing, in German, that he would ignore the teachings of Hippocrates and Galen and would instead demonstrate the truths of disease from his own experience. To emphasize the point, he cast a book of Galen's writings and Avicenna's *Canon* onto a students' bonfire booming, as he did so, with typical modesty:

"The buckles of my shoes know more of medicine than both of these venerable physicians together! All the universities and all the authorities in the world know less than the hairs of my beard!"

This was greeted with shouts and raucous applause as his beard was sparse in the extreme and he was, indeed, reputed to be a eunuch.

Unabashed, he continued:

"*I* am the true monarch of medicine. You will follow *me*. You, Avicenna; you, Galen; you, Rhazes. You will follow *me*, you messieurs of Paris, of Montpellier, you meinen Herren of Cologne, of Vienna, and all, however many you may be; you who inhabit the isles of the sea; you Italians, Dalmatians, Athenians; you Greek, you Arab, you Jew, follow *me*, your king!"

I stood with the crowd, recording his words.

"The humours of Hippocrates and Galen do not cause disease. They do not exist! – but if they did..." the contempt in his voice invited challenge; he waited. There was only silence. His audience was stunned; that any man should have the gall even to harbour such heretical thoughts, let alone proclaim them publicly. "...if they did, they would be the consequences and not the causes of disease.

"A crowd of physicians rise up against me," he roared – and that, at least, was indisputable. "They give you the names: bile, melancholy, phlegm and blood. But who has seen bile in Nature? How can phlegm resemble one of the elements? How does blood resemble air? You say *this* is a vice of the blood, and that of the liver; but what, I pray you, has given you the eyes of a lynx that you know so well that the blood or the liver is the cause when you are utterly ignorant of the nature of the blood?

"Instead of saying *this* is due to bile, *that* to melancholy, we should say this is due to arsenic, *that* to alum and, also, *this* is under the influence of Saturn, *that* of Mars. Thus you can see that half the disease comes from the earth and half from the heavens. Again, you say that the disease is due to the blood – but the blood is no more than wood, and just as there are many kinds of wood, so there are many kinds of blood. And just as the heavens send the trees to sleep in winter and wake them in summer, so the blood similarly changes with the seasons.

"From this it follows that a physician should say that *this* disease is turpentine, *that* is mountain celery, the *other* is hellebore, and not *this* is phlegm, *that* is rheum, a coryza, a catarrh. Those names have no medical foundation."

[If, Dr Annandale, you regard Oporinus's tale as showing how Paracelsus employed destructive criticism so that he could then indulge in ridicule, we might admire him for his defiance and questioning of ancient authority. But alas! since he firmly believed that disease *did* originate partly in the stars, and since he plumbed the depths of absurdity with his doctrines, I have abbreviated Oporinus's account which fully occupied a week of our journey.]

I was compelled by a sense of duty to record all that Paracelsus said, despite my conviction that most of it was worthless (Oporinus continued). He had concocted three important doctrines – the entities, the archaeus and the tartarian or calculous origins of disease. But, since consistency was not one of his virtues, each of these could be the sole cause of disease, depending on which suited his fancy. He stated that since there were five entities (to which, true to his inconsistent reasoning, he gave Latin names), and since all diseases were produced by them, there must be five phlegms, five hydropathies, five jaundices, five fevers, five cancers and five of every disease known to man.

The archaeus was the invention of a Benedictine monk some fifty years previously. It was not so much the soul as a form of deity that lived at the entrance to the stomach from where it directed and, by chemical means, regulated the bodily functions. Death came with its loss.

But, when the mood took him, the very same diseases could be produced only by tartar. Every moisture on earth had, so he said, a substance within it that was prone to coagulate. Wine, on keeping, coagulates and the clot separates and adheres to the side of the vessel. Water contains a tartar which separates on boiling and adheres to the side of the kettle. Urine contains a tartar which separates as stones in the kidney or bladder. Bile contains a tartar which separates to form gallstones. Blood contains a tartar which separates as a blood clot.

Paracelsus passed like a destructive hurricane through medical authority, denying the demigods of the past and contradicting his illustrious contemporaries, whatever they said. The apothecaries and the herbalists, already in conflict with the alchemists, also felt the sting of his influence. At the moment when new and exotic botanicals were flooding in from the Americas, the alchemists decided they had more chance of finding a medical remedy among the residues in their retorts than of turning base metal into gold. Into the fray stepped Paracelsus, his philosophy resting on chemical principles first set out by that same Benedictine monk who had conjured up the archaeus. There were apparently three primary substances, but they were philosophical substances rather than chemical elements: philosophical sulphur, philosophical mercury and philosophical salt (this last being the state of equilibrium between the other two). They were operated by the spiritual force of the archaeus. [Make of this what you will, Dr Annandale.]

He was a fervent advocate of tinctures amongst which he favoured his *Lilium Paracelsi,* a concoction prepared from alloys of antimony* and iron, antimony and tin and antimony and copper. [How much of his success as a physician depended on the alcoholic content of these tinctures, I leave you, Dr Annandale, to decide!]

When I worked with him he always kept several preparations stewing on his furnaces – for example, a sublimate of oil of arsenic, a mixture of saffron and iron or his marvellous Opodeloch, a plaster. I cannot recall him ever giving any recommendations about diet or hygiene. To his credit, though, he was bitterly opposed to polypharmacy – the

---

* The fact that antimony is a dangerous poison did not dim Paracelsus's enthusiasm for the metal. Its use as a drug was, indeed, subsequently banned though the prohibition could be circumvented by giving white wine in cups made of antimony. In modern times compounds of antimony, such as tartar emetic, have been used in the treatment of schistosomiasis. – J.G.

treatment with many drugs together.

His popularity among those who sought his help was due in no small measure to his ability to tell them what they wanted to hear. To the religious, he declared that his system was based on Holy Scripture – the Bible was the key to his theory of disease, which was founded on the Apocalypse. He proclaimed himself to be a man who submitted without a second thought to the Divine Will; who identified himself with the celestial intelligencies; who possessed the philosophers' stone; who could cure every ill and who could prolong his life at will, and all because he possessed the tincture which had been used by Adam and the Patriarchs before the Deluge to prolong their lives for eight or nine centuries.

To the sceptic, he professed the grossest pantheism. To the credulous, he posed as a magician (for magic is a highly refined area of knowledge): he had received letters from Galen and had visited Avicenna at the Gates of Hell. He duped them with his accounts of drinkable gold, the philosophers' stone, the quintessence, the mithridate and whatever else entered his mind at the given moment.

* * *

"Eventually, having been driven from city to city by his ungovernable delight in irritating authority," Oporinus came to the end of his tale, "Paracelsus was offered the ecclesiastical protection of Archbishop Ernst of Salzburg. He accepted, but a few months later he was killed in a drunken brawl. As the prophet Jeremiah truly said, 'Can the Aethiopian change his skin, or the leopard his spots?' "

Oporinus walked on in silence with an arm laid thoughtfully across the neck of one of the animals.

"You know," he said, as if the idea had just come to him, "had it not been for Paracelsus we would not be making this journey today."

I looked at him in amazement. What possible connection could there be between that unscrupulous charlatan and these invaluable woodcuts?

"For all that his teachings were unmitigated claptrap," Oporinus was responding to my incredulity in his own way, "he left the world a different place from the one he had entered. Although he would never forgive me for saying so, his studies on chemistry, concealed by the cloak of alchemy, have expanded the scope of medical therapy. Since his death, many physicians have been persuaded of the absurdities of alchemy and have turned to chemicals* in a more reasoned – though not necessarily effective – manner. No, wait!" He thought I was about to interrupt at the seeming irrelevance of his words, but my reaction had quite another cause. At last I realized what Telesphorus had meant when he said that alchemy – though, more precisely, an alchemist – would open a new sphere of medical knowledge.

"Paracelsus has had a two-fold effect on medicine – intellectual and practical. If I had begun with the intellectual, I should probably have had difficulty convincing you. So, I deliberately drew your attention to his practical influence on pharmacy – of which I imagine you are already aware – in the hope of thus making you receptive to the abstruseness of the intellectual influence.

"The teachings of Hippocrates, Aristotle and Galen were – and, to many, still are – regarded as divinely inspired and containing the full sum of medical knowledge. Consequently nothing remains to be discovered. That is why scholars have been searching for original Greek texts, to prepare fresh translations uncluttered by the detritus and distortions of the intervening ages. These ancient texts hold the key to the eternal truths. The only path to progress lies in their rediscovery and reinterpretation. Until Paracelsus arrived to trouble the waters!

"He may have failed, in his own eyes, to make the walls of authority fall down flat by his relentless trumpeting, but his questioning and ridiculing of the teachings of the great have created a breach ready for storming. Ridicule, you know, is a wonderful weapon for it creates a vulnerability to serious attack. Although he died as ignominiously as he had lived, he was not struck down by the heavens for his iniquity, and this gave strength to others themselves to challenge the received truth. Without Paracelsus before him, Vesalius would never have dared to publish his anatomical discoveries – and we would not be travelling this road."

[You, Dr Annandale, may find the reverence with which those three greats of the ancient world were held, to be beyond belief. But think on this: Averroës long ago asserted that Aristotle's doctrine was "the perfection of truth, and his understanding attained the utmost limit of human ability; so that it might be truly said of him that he was created

---

* Minerals (as distinct from botanicals) had been used in the past, but in the main for external application – astringents, ointments and the like. Traditional humoral medicine had relied on herbals. – J.G.

and given to the world by Divine Providence that we might see in him how much it is possible for a man to know." There were dons in your grandfather's time at the University of Oxford who might well have said – and believed – those very words!]

When we had reached Basle and the woodcuts had been safely entrusted to the printing house, I lodged with Oporinus. He was a most knowledgeable and agreeable companion who needed little urging to talk.

"What I was saying about Paracelsus liberating the medical mind accounts only in part for the existence of Vesalius's anatomy. The intense intellectual energy investing all aspects of human activity today has taken longer to reach medicine than some other spheres. But the scholars in these spheres had, in their time, also accepted the books of antiquity as their supreme authority and had neither the desire nor the means to improve upon them. Until, that is, something awoke them to the arrival, in a changing world, of the truly scientific spirit*. In the military field that something was gunpowder. In art, it was a less explosive occurrence," he grinned. "It had started with Giotto..." my heart leapt "...who painted his saints as real people and not in the stylized Gothic form.

"My friend, are you ill? Have I distressed you?" Oporinus was concerned as he had noticed my agitation – indeed, he could scarcely have failed to do so, since my hand shook violently as I rested my tankard on the table.

"No, no, I assure you I am well." In spite of myself my voice trembled like my hand. "Your mention of Giotto brought to mind a romantic adventure I had a few years ago in Assisi with a delightful young lady." My emotions took refuge in understatement. "It ended tragically with her sudden death. But, please, I beg of you, continue."

Much to my relief, however, he left me alone while he descended to his cellars to refill the jug. By the time he returned – and I suspect he had kept himself tactfully occupied – I had ceased my weeping at my memories of Fiammetta. With my encouragement, this time he continued. I was at last, it seemed, to learn how an artist could have an influence on medicine.

* Oporinus is here referring to the scientific spirit in what we would now regard as its modern sense: the acquisition of knowledge by observation and experiment, its critical evaluation and its organization under general principles. Self-evidently, it differed from any "science" that had preceded it, as this had been dependent on "divine inspiration" of one sort or another. – J.G.

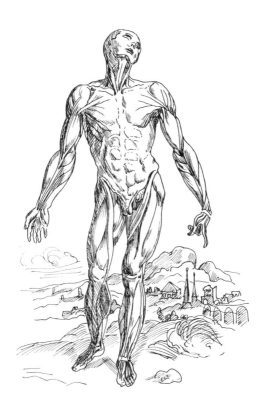

For five years Vesalius dissected and Calcar drew. Dissection of the superficial muscles from Vesalius's Fabrica*.*

"On our journey, I was speaking as a Greek scholar and amanuensis to Paracelsus. Now, I shall talk as a typographer and, in my own way, an artist. The freeing of the intellect combined with two other driving forces has unleashed the scientific spirit of medicine in the shape of this book by Vesalius and Calcar.

"In the past, anatomies were necessarily demonstrations, since anatomists had little or no idea how they should record their work pictorially. Thus their drawings were symbolic, fulfilling spiritual needs rather than the requirements of realism. And, after Galen, the anatomy seen and recorded at dissections was unalterably Galen's.

"You, Balthasar, I believe followed Vesalius for five years while he dissected and Calcar drew*. We both know that Calcar's woodcuts are lifelike representations of the structures Vesalius demonstrated to his audiences. Yet Galenists still maintain that the drawings are inaccurate. Sylvius even tried to make Vesalius recant some of his teachings – and this despite his own valuable service to anatomy by ridding it of mongrel Arabic terms and returning to the Latin of ancient writers such as Celsus**. Vesalius had been a student under Sylvius in Paris, and it is ironic that the Latin nomenclature helped give much-needed precision to his demonstrations and Calcar's drawings.

"This, the ability to represent accurately what is seen during dissection, is the first of the driving forces I mentioned; the second is the ability to disseminate that information. I believe it to be true that without our artists and without our printing houses – and without the heretical Paracelsus – anatomy might never have freed itself from ancient authority. Anatomists would continue to see what Galen had said they would see."

"So," I said, to indicate I had overcome my emotional lapse, "once Giotto had broken free from the spell of Gothic art, anatomists could give a true representation of their dissections?"

"No, not immediately," Oporinus answered. "In my imagination I see Giotto holding open the gate through which Masaccio would pass a hundred years later. Giotto brought painting to life and Masaccio gave it space – his vision of reality was a function of his mind as well as of his eye; his vision of space was his intellectual vision of reality."

"All in keeping with the spirit of the times." I felt some comment was called for, although I was not entirely sure what he meant.

"Yes, particularly as the vision was not entirely of his own creation," Oporinus continued, apparently oblivious to my incomprehension. "Brunelleschi had slipped through a nearby 'gate' in Florence a few years previously. In his work as an architect, he had conceived the principle of perspective for the rational distribution of architectural elements in space. Masaccio had the genius to see how this could be applied to painting: he used the laws of perspective to create the

*Although Vesalius was professor of anatomy at Padua, during those five years he also dissected and lectured at Bologna and Pisa. – J.G.
** This Latin nomenclature is familiar today – and not only to anatomists. – J.G.

conditions for perfect unity of time and place, thus eliminating all inessentials*." This was indeed the artist in Oporinus talking!

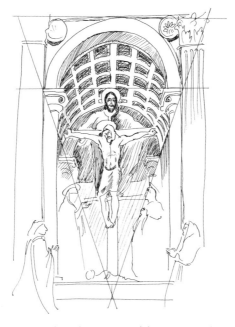

Fresco of The Holy Trinity with St John, St Mary and the Two Donors (c.1425) *in Santa Maria Novella, by Masaccio, who used the laws of perspective to create the conditions for perfect unity of time and space. He discovered the vanishing point which is dictated by the angle of the receding object (in this case, the lower edge of the barrrel-vaulted ceiling, indicated by the ruled lines).*

"Once Masaccio had shown the way, artists began to pour through Giotto's 'gate' to explore the new world before them. Artistic activity was equated with science – based either on geometry and mathematics, which gave a logical explanation of the structure of the universe, or on the direct methodological study of nature. The artists studied, drew and painted the human body; but without a knowledge of its structure, they could not achieve a true representation. So they began to dissect

* Probably the best examples are the frescos in Santa Maria del Carmine in Florence, painted by Masaccio in 1427, the year before his untimely death. His most significant achievement as regards perspective was his discovery of the vanishing point. – J.G.

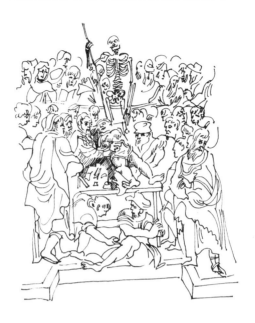

Detail from the frontispiece of Vesalius's De humani corporis fabrica *showing Vesalius dissecting.*

for themselves whenever the opportunity offered and to draw what they saw unencumbered by Galenic preconceptions of the anatomy they would uncover.

"When a great anatomist, like Vesalius, works with a great artist, like Calcar, the repercussions will resound down the ages. You, Paolo, a physician, will say that the palm should be awarded to Vesalius, but I, speaking as an artist, would award it to Calcar for, without him and Giotto and Masaccio before him, Vesalius's dissections would have suffered the same fate as that of all his predecessors. Furthermore – and I now speak as a typographer – I would award the palm to Gutenberg who showed how it was possible to print from moveable metal type. Without him, both your Vesalius and my Calcar would still be dependent on books prepared laboriously in manuscript."

*   *   *

While artists had poured through Giotto's 'gate', anatomists more slowly climbed the 'stile' provided by Vesalius. Galen's intellectual hold continued to dominate the mind despite the evidence of the senses.

Before anatomists dared to publish a discovery that contradicted his word, they felt impelled to secure their position by repeated and emphatic demonstrations before witnesses of unimpeachable honesty.

Shortly after his book* was published, Vesalius travelled round the universities of Europe in an attempt to convert his critics – his enemies, he called them – by demonstrating the new anatomy. When he returned to Padua, his reception was so venomous in its intensity that, in utter disgust, he burnt all his notebooks and accepted the appointment (almost a sinecure) of court physician to the Holy Roman Emperor, Charles V and, subsequently, to Charles's son, Philip II of Spain. He was content with this life for twenty years until the day he received a copy of a text by Fallopio – one of his former students and now occupying his old chair of anatomy at Padua – in which many of his own errors had been corrected. And, as he soon learnt, other former students were making discoveries that had escaped him. Anatomy was no dead subject; the time had come for him to return to the dissecting table.

But it was not to be.

Telesphorus appeared, as if from nowhere, with the news that Vesalius had died in a shipwreck on his way back from the Holy Land.

"You know," Telesphorus said, "it was the man's anatomical honesty that I admire most. Can you remember what he said to you on one occasion when he had finished discussing the Emperor's health?"

I could indeed. "When I first dissected the heart," he had said, "I could find no evidence of the pores between the ventricles that Galen had described so graphically. Yet I was reluctant to deny their existence as how else were we to explain the flow of blood. I simply wrote of my wonderment at a God who could give us an invisible passage for the blood. But, when I revised the book in later years, I knew there were no pores and I said so in quite explicit terms. Do you wonder that the Galenists hate me?"

I believe he knew that by his confidence in rejecting the pores to which Galen had ascribed an otherwise inexplicable function, he had revealed the existence of yet another new world lying beyond his chosen one of anatomy.

---

* *De humani corporis fabrica*. Basel: Oporinus, 1543 (Second edition, 1555). The book is commonly known as the *Fabrica*. – J.G.

14

"I began to think that the blood might have a certain movement, as it were, in a circle" *

I t was not what he had discovered, but how he had arrived there that the old man was remembering for his questioner.

"I thought the blood must move in a circle when I noticed that the valves in the veins of so many parts of the body were so placed as to give free passage of blood towards the heart, but to oppose its passage in the opposite direction," was William Harvey's response to Robert Boyle's opening question.

For a moment, in my mind's eye, I was back with Vesalius a hundred years ago, listening to his friend, Canano from Ferrara, describe the membranes – as he called them – in the veins which, he said, prevented the backward flow of blood. Vesalius, though, believed the membranes were there simply to strengthen the veins, and this belief was generally accepted as it did not compromise Galenic thinking.

In the years between, I had travelled leisurely around the universities of Europe watching anatomists reap where Vesalius had sown. They explored the depths of the body and various were the tubes, ducts and canals named in honour of their discoverers. I have no doubt that my presence at the right university at the right time was not fortuitous but due to Telesphorus's guiding hand. He led me first to Amatus Lusitanus who spoke of ostiola (or little doors) in the veins that prevented the return of blood – just like those in the heart, a point that Canano had

---

* Harvey realizes that the blood circulates. Second half of the 16th to the first half of the 17th century. – J.G.

also made.

But Galen was still a power in the land. Indeed, Vesalius's convincing demonstration that the pores between the ventricles did not exist was attributed by some to their natural disappearance after death and by others to a change in man's anatomy since Galen! It was this baleful influence that was preventing men's minds from realizing the functional implications of the new anatomy.

This was all too apparent when Telesphorus decided we should make another visit to Padua where the chair of anatomy was occupied by Fabricius. I arrived bearing a letter of introduction purporting to be from Cesalpino who had recently published his speculation* that in systole the heart sent blood into the aorta and pulmonary artery and, in diastole, received it back again through the venae cavae and pulmonary veins (the opposite to received opinion). The letter was, in fact, one of the concoctions Telesphorus had devised as a means of "giving me a recent past", and they were invariably effective.

Fabricius glanced at the letter, saw it was from Pope Clement's personal physician and embraced me warmly.

"Come, Paolo, you have arrived opportunely. You shall be of the first to bear witness to a discovery which thrusts anatomy into a new field. We anatomists must now go beyond a description of what we find and determine the *function* of anatomical structures and the *purpose* of that function. For Nature does nothing without a purpose."

His flow of words was uninterrupted while, taking me by the arm, he walked me to the anatomy theatre he had had built at his own expense. I knew it to be large but I did not expect to find its interior windowless. Fabricius dissected by the light of candles, demonstrating as he did so to the students crowding the balconies rising perpendicularly above him.

While he dissected he continued to talk, as much for my benefit as for that of the students. It was the same old story: Galen teaches that arterial blood carries the vital pneuma to every part of the body where it is almost completely consumed; it does not return to the heart; it is the carrier of life. Venous blood ebbs and flows to meet the needs of the tissues for nourishment. [The variations on this theme down the

---

* *Quaestionum peripateticarum, libri* V. Venetiis: apud Iuntas, 1571. This "discovery" of both the systemic and the pulmonary circulations has been rejected – except in Italy – since it lacked the support of experimental evidence. – J.G.

ages, Dr Annandale, are almost as numerous as the anatomists themselves – and as the medical historians of your day!]

Fabricius directed his assistant to throw the candlelight more clearly on the vein in the leg he had been dissecting. He had laid it open.

"Here you see my ostiola within the vein. They quite evidently hinder the outward flow of blood. They do not impede its inward flow. This is their function. But what is the purpose of that function?" He looked up and around. No one was prepared to offer an answer.

"No? Then I shall have to tell you. These ostiola function like the floodgates that obstruct the flow of water in the sluices of a mill. Their purpose is to prevent the blood from flooding the extremities of the body. Galen said that an attractive force served this purpose. But I have shown it to be a visible anatomical structure!"

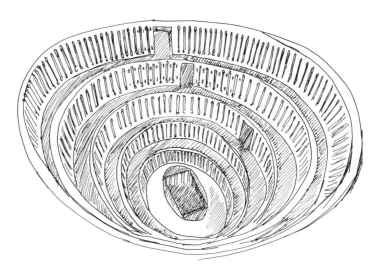

The anatomy theatre at Padua that Fabricius built at his own expense. Since the interior was windowless, he dissected by the light of candles.

Fabricius had thus opened the way to a mechanistic, as opposed to a Galenic, physiological explanation. Nevertheless, it was one that was quite acceptable to Galenic authority as it contradicted none of Galen's basic assumptions. Even so he waited twenty-nine years before publishing his "discovery"*. However, during those years Saloman Alberti had published his *Tres orationes* in which he had illustrated the valvulis, as he called them, and had drawn attention to their one-way action.

I shook myself free of my daydreaming to hear Harvey explain to Boyle how he had learnt of the existence of the venous valves.

"I spent the first two years of the century in Padua, studying medicine and anatomy under Fabricius. It was he who inspired me to devote my mind to function and purpose rather than structure. And he it was, too, who impressed on me the importance of the valves. Both in Padua and on my return to London, I made frequent dissections of human and animal bodies. Observing the heart in the living animal was fraught with difficulty owing to the rapidity of the movement which in many animals remained visible but for the wink of an eye and the length of a lightning flash. I answered this by studying the slow-moving hearts of cold-blooded animals and of dying dogs and pigs.

"In none of these dissections was it possible to show the pores that Galen supposed to lie between the ventricles. Moreover, I was unable to find evidence for the existence of vital pneuma or psychic pneuma. I tell you that when philosophers and physicians discuss the role of these spirits in the workings of the body, they are making an unworthy attempt to veil their ignorance."

He paused for a moment or two while he gathered himself to continue with the matter in hand.

"I also read widely and was assiduous in confirming or confuting the anatomical findings of others. Of particular relevance to your questions, Dr Boyle," Harvey looked up from the notes he held on his lap and nodded at Dr Boyle, "I repeated the experiments of Colombo on the passage of blood through the lungs** and confirmed that it was so."

"But," Boyle interrupted, "what made you reject your old teacher's explanation of the purpose of the valves? After all, you were – you are – a respected member of the medical fraternity. You had already been

---

* *De venarum ostiolis.* Patavii: Laurentij Pasquati, 1603. Fabricius also published the first account of the development of the chick embryo since Aristotle. – J.G.

** *De re anatomica.* Venetiis: Nicolai Benilacquae, 1559. Colombo was almost certainly familiar with the *Christianismi restitutio* of the French physician and theologian, Michael Servetus (1511-1553), which contains an account of the pulmonary circulation. Publication of this work led to Servetus's death at the stake in Geneva, copies of the book being used to start the bonfire. Fewer than a handful survived. – J.G.

Lumleian lecturer at the College of Physicians for thirteen years and three times one of the Censors of the College when you published *De motu cordis**. And yet you must have known your work would have a harmful effect on the traditional medicine of which you were a part."

On the table at Harvey's side were his old lecture notes and a copy of *De motu cordis*, to both of which he had referred from time to time. He picked up the book.

"If you turn to chapter eight you will see that I have kept faith with Aristotle." He leant across the table and handed the opened book to Boyle. "I shall return to that example in due time, but throughout I have been true to his philosophy. There is nothing revolutionary about my work."

I had been watching his face as he spoke and those last words were sincere and without a taint of false modesty.

"You will also see that in my lecture notes," he pushed these across the table, "I referred to the venous membranes as valves, not as ostiola, as Fabricius would have done. By naming them thus, the idea that they closed completely, or almost so, is established in the mind. I believe it was this matter of nomenclature that prevented Fabricius from discovering their true purpose. His book contains a drawing of the opened heart to show the cusps of the aortic valve which he likened to the ostiola of the veins – the sole obvious difference being that the aortic valve has three cusps whereas the venous valves have only two or one. He knew the aortic valve permitted flow in one direction only, yet the similarity of purpose of the venous valves escaped him."

Harvey laid his left palm flat on the table. The veins on the back of the old man's hand stood out quite clearly. He pressed on one of them with the index finger of his right hand and ran the nail of the thumb back along the vein towards his wrist. The vein collapsed, leaving a hollow channel until it reached a valve. When he removed his index finger the vein refilled.

"A very simple demonstration that the venous valves prevent the backward flow of blood. In my original experiments, though, I used the forearm with a tourniquet to distend the veins, as you will see illustrated in the book. I first wrapped a length of cloth tightly around the arm

* *Exercitatio anatomica de motu cordis ex sanguinis in animalibus.* Francofurti: Guilelmi Fitzeri, 1628. Commonly referred to as *De motu cordis*. – J.G.

above the elbow to stop the flow of blood in the arteries, then I loosened it sufficiently to restore arterial flow, but not the flow in the veins. These swelled up, so demonstrating to me that a connection must exist between the two in the extremities.

"I was greatly impressed also by the abundance of these valves. Surely, I reasoned, if in some places the valves did not act with perfect accuracy, their greater number plainly served to prevent the passage of blood

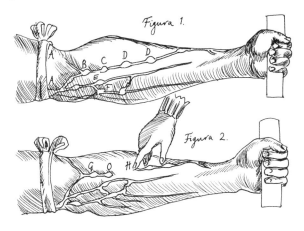

In his original experiments Harvey distended the veins of the forearm by the use of a tourniquet to demonstrate that the venous valves prevented the backward flow of blood.

from the centre. Moreover, the existence of valves in the jugular veins, also preventing flow backwards from the centre, was contrary to Fabricius's idea of their purpose. And, let me add, there are no valves in the arteries save at their exits from the heart."

"So, a year or two after you had prepared your notes for the Lumleian lectures on anatomy* you had already decided that the blood moved with a circular motion?" Boyle enquired. "And yet you added nothing about your discovery for another eight or so years, although you made many other additions to the notebook."

"I believe you would have done the same." Harvey's answer was plainly matter-of-fact. "The content of the lectures was so arranged

* *Prelectiones anatomiae universalis.* 1616. – J.G.

that the full course took six years to complete. At first, I had only the evidence of the valves to present; the physiological argument to replace the old teaching was still inadequate. Then, when I had gathered a sufficiency of evidence, I was writing my book and there was no need to insert more than a brief mention in the notebook for the next occasion when I should deliver that lecture. Nor did I trouble to correct statements that I believed were now erroneous."

Harvey leant back in his chair and closed his eyes. His notes slid to the floor.

"There is not much more to tell," he overcame his weariness and continued. "After many dissections on the living, I saw clearly that the symmetry and magnitude of the ventricles of the heart and of the vessels entering and leaving it were too large for their supposed purpose. Nature, who does nothing in vain, would not have needlessly given them such a large size. How was I to explain this unless the purpose was to transmit blood in great quantity – far greater than the small amount hitherto supposed to originate from the liver. Furthermore, my investigations led me to observe that this great quantity was transmitted in so short a time.

"Thus I have written," and he pointed across the table to *De motu cordis* lying in Boyle's hands. "Privately I began to think that the blood might have a certain movement, as it were, in a circle.

"So, Dr Boyle, I shall draw together the strings of our conversation, if you will pass me my book." He opened it, found the page he wanted and began reading.

" 'By reason and experiment I have shown that, by the beat of the ventricles, blood flows through the lungs and heart and is pumped to the whole body. There it passes through pores in the flesh' " (shades of Galen, I thought, this is the one flaw in his argument that he should have to conjure up "pores" to account for what he cannot explain) " 'into veins through which it returns from everywhere in the periphery to the centre – from the smaller veins into the larger ones, finally coming to the vena cava and right atrium.

" 'This occurs in such an amount, with such an outflow through the arteries, and such a reflux through the veins, that it cannot be supplied by the food consumed. It is also much more than is needed for nourishment. We must therefore conclude that the blood in the animal body moves around in a circle continuously, and that the purpose of the heart is to accomplish this by pumping. This is the only reason for the motion and beat of the heart.' "

He closed the book, replaced it on the table, patted it lovingly and begged to take his leave. As he stood up, I was struck once again by how short a man he was.

When he had seen Harvey into the care of his servant, Boyle returned.

"Harvey, as you know, has not been without his critics. The most vehement of his attackers has been the Parisian, Riolan – as you might expect of the man." Boyle was happy to talk about Harvey and I made a willing listener. "Riolan sees Harvey's proof that the blood is in circular motion as a threat to his reputation and practice which is strongly founded in Galenic medicine; you would have to travel a great distance to find a more ardent disciple. Having been, with reluctance, compelled to accept the existence of a circulation, he now states that the heart pumps no more than a drop or two with each beat. Then, having estimated how many drops are pumped in the hour, he has calculated that there can only be two or three circulations each day. To explain Harvey's findings, he has resorted to the popular refuge of the intellectually destitute Galenists: changes after death! As the heart of the dying animal slows, the blood accumulates and the heart appears to pump these greater quantities. This compromise allows him to continue teaching a Galenic form of physiology according to which he can still argue that blood is produced by the liver*.

"For reasons, perhaps on account of some obscure French logic, Riolan also objects to Harvey's concept of two circulations. So, in the letters he is writing to the Frenchman, Harvey is delighting in pointing out that there are, in fact, three circulations, the third being..." Boyle searched through the papers on his table, found what he wanted and began reading: "...'a very short circulation, namely from the left ventricle to the right, driving a portion of the blood round through the coronary arteries and veins, which are distributed with their small branches through the walls and septum of the heart.' These are notes of a conversation I had with Harvey concerning his reply to Riolan,"

---

* In 1673, Louis XIV established a professorial chair to which he appointed Pierre Dionis (d.1718) to run a course of anatomical dissection with lectures at which the true nature was to be taught. The King thus overruled the medical establishment. – J.G.

he added in explanation.

"The undeniable truth of Harvey's work is founded on experimentation and observation and not on what is to be found in books. He refuses to accept what others have written until he has confirmed it for himself. Even so," Boyle hesitated a moment and looked at me, as if assessing how I might respond – it was a look I had come to know well over the years – "even so Harvey is unwilling to let go of the past. Despite his contention that the heart is merely a pump, he believes it to be driven by the pulsative power of the soul; he rejects completely the mechanical and chemical concepts of nature that are gaining in popularity today. Truly, if any man may be said to stand at a crossroads, it is William Harvey!"

Boyle was showing me out of his lodgings when an idea seemed to come to him. "Should you wish to know more about the mechanistic concept," he said, "I would advise you to visit Descartes – he is somewhere in the Low Countries. His philosophical approach is, however, quite the reverse of Harvey's. While Harvey draws his conclusions from meticulous observations, Descartes first constructs a clear picture in his mind and then verifies, or not, this mental concept by experimental observation. But beware, for he is inclined to select only those facts which fit his theories!"

On which encouraging note we bade each other farewell.

*   *   *

"So, Paolo Balthasar, you have come from England?" was Descartes's abrupt greeting; he treasured his privacy and preferred not to receive visitors. "From London? And did you meet William Harvey?"

"Yes," I replied. Before I could continue, Descartes was talking again. That, he enjoyed when he could expound his own philosophies.

"I agree with him that the blood moves around the body in a circular manner, but not with his explanation of the driving force of the heart, since this is not in tune with mechanistic principles. You must understand that the body is a machine which is fired by the innate heat of the heart. This heat vapourizes the blood and causes the heart to expand and to drive particles of blood into the arteries."

[Even though his physiology of the circulation may have been worthless, Dr Annandale, Descartes's analogy of the workings of the body with those of a machine was valuable – and probably inevitable in an age of mechanical invention – in that it undermined the thinking that the bodily functions were driven by the soul (or souls). In succeeding generations the analogy shifted to whatever was the popular science of the time – from mechanics, through chemistry to the electronics of your day. The difference from Descartes is that in later years these analogies were validated experimentally. The body is the union of them all, with probably sciences yet to be discovered.]

We were sitting in the scrubbed cleanliness of his Dutch home in the quietly dignified city of Amsterdam and, probably owing to the warmth – for he was averse to cold – I was finding it difficult to concentrate sufficiently to follow his thesis.

"You are perplexed?" he enquired. "Then let me take you through my philosophy of the body's functions.

"At the beginning, you must free your mind from the notions of humours, elements and qualities so beloved of the ancients. Instead, accept that the body is governed by mechanistic laws. It, like the world we live in, is matter in motion."

Descartes's reputation as a mathematician was already well known to me. His excessive love of the subject was, perhaps, not surprising, as it was the only science that could be depended on with certainty – and Descartes was determined to apply it to every aspect of learning or, seemingly, to die in the attempt. In some instances, he succeeded, in others he failed. But, watching and listening to the man, I knew why his philosophy of life was doomed to be unworkable – it was his denial of human emotions, spirituality, of the essential quality that makes a human being a human being, call it what you will.

"Now," and he rose and began pacing up and down. "Now, matter and mind both emanate from the same divine source and operate along parallel lines, but *they are unrelated*." He spoke those last words with dramatic emphasis.

I then realized how he had managed to escape the wrath of the theologians for so long: he had been careful to write nothing that could be construed as in direct contradiction to the first chapter of Genesis. Alas! the heresy seekers had eventually decided that he was using science as a cover for an attack on religion and had proceeded to denounce him as an enemy of the Christian faith. Fortunately, the Estates General in the Low Countries had refused to surrender him to Papal authority – as was their practice for all who enjoyed their hospitality – and he was able to continue his work.

"The soul," he proceeded to explain, "which is situated in the pineal gland in the brain, can call forth no movement unless all the bodily organs which are needed for that movement are properly disposed. Nevertheless, when the body already has all its organs properly arranged for a particular movement, it has no need of the soul to carry this out. Hence all movement except those which we know to depend upon thought ought not to be attributed to the soul, but to the mere disposition of organs."

[He spoke, as he wrote, with deliberate obfuscation – to blind his enemies with science, as you, Dr Annandale, might say? I think I saw what he was getting at. At least it was better than his belief that the nerves were hollow tubes designed to transmit the juice of animal spirit to all parts of the body and that they contained valves. (Did he, I wonder, copy this idea of valves from Harvey's work?) Nevertheless, in his beliefs about movement you can discern a parallel with your voluntary (central and peripheral) and involuntary (autonomic) nervous systems.]

I visited him frequently endeavouring to comprehend his physiological ideas. But they were entangled in Galenic thinking and he remained essentially a Galenist to the end – an end which was not very far away.

One day as summer was mellowing into autumn, he announced he would be leaving for Sweden. He had been invited by Queen Christina to initiate her into the mysteries of higher mathematics and philosophy. It was destined to be his last journey, as that strange queen had a habit of conversing in her unheated library in the early hours of the morning. Descartes caught a chill at the end of January and died early in February from a congestion of the lungs.

15

The circle is completed by the science of microscopy *

here is a garden in Bologna – I hope it is still there, restored to its former glory by some loving hand – lying close under the city wall. The house is invisible from the arbour where I spend my days, alone with my thoughts.

I have lived here for some time now and have adopted the life of a recluse. My sole pleasure is to tend my herb garden and prepare medicines which Telesphorus distributes to the sick poor. I seek, not to sustain the therapeutic authority of Galenism which flags in the face of competition from Paracelsian chemical remedies (often given as Christian charity – to the intense annoyance of the commercial herbalists), but to ensure a fair balance of choice for the people of Bologna. My herbals, being a part of the tried and tested traditions of the land, are especially popular with travellers from the countryside.

The garden is surrounded by an ancient wall – that of the city forming one boundary only – with every nook and crevice adorned with the colour of its sweet-scented occupant. Above the entrance is a horse's head carved in stone, an ancient Roman spur to all that grows within to be fruitful. And carved above the door to my physic garden is an open rose surmounted by two buds, a device to protect the secrets of the herbalists' art. I shall not betray those secrets, except to say that my garden is a confusion of scents, with first one and then another

*The beginning of microscopic anatomy. Second half of the 17th century. – J.G.

predominating as I wander, dreaming, along the paths, sometimes adding to the intensity of the odours as a careless foot crushes an errant plant thrusting up between the flagstones.

I think that in those years I was at the lowest ebb of my life. I was beyond despair; I was trembling on the borders of madness, and that would never do as, to their considerable displeasure, it would cheat the gods of their full payment. It is said that a man is closer to his god in a garden than anywhere else on earth. This I knew and had experienced many times. But in Bologna, I was strangely unsettled. Yes, I was at peace among my flowers and they brought me comfort, but not the comfort of the human embrace that would heal my soul. Were my gods, then, slipping away from me? (I still believed in my ancient gods, the gods of Nature. I could not wholly accept those that seemed to me to be the creations of the human mind.) Worse – for I placed love above *all* the gods – was Ishtar slipping away? I tried desperately to conjure her up, to picture her tending the flowers, planning and planting for the coming seasons far better than ever I could. If I had her in my arms, I would be closer to my gods, I would be *with* them in very Paradise. But condemned as I myself was to what now seemed the certainty of everlasting life on earth, Paradise had to remain a dream, for I could never condemn her to share such a fate.

At this moment in my misery, Telesphorus appeared, bringing refreshment to lull me into sleep through the heat of the afternoon.

"Telesphorus." I paused while he sat himself cross-legged on the warm grass. "You know I do not ask why things happen to me. I have long learnt to accept that what the gods choose to do with me is inevitable and unalterable. But tell me why I feel my mind is about to break. I have this unbearable ache for Ishtar, yet I know she is not in this world. I cannot bring her presence to mind and I have no sense that she is about to return. Has she given me such pleasure that I must now pay the price by losing her for ever?" I had difficulty controlling the agony in my voice.

Telesphorus leant forward and took my hand. I felt a surge of spiritual strength pass from his small body to mine. "No, Bal-sarra-uzur. Keep faith; she will never desert you." He smiled. "Your destinies are linked into eternity. But regrettably Trithemius's experiment has disturbed the even pattern of events and now for a while I cannot predict the precise moment of her return. Yet remember that when in the past she has been away, I have woven a spell of forgetfulness around you."

"I also have a sense of disillusion over the advancement taking place in our learning." Although I knew Telesphorus was aware of all that troubled me, I felt a desperate need to unburden my soul. "Vesalius and Harvey may have added immeasurably to our understanding of anatomy and of the manner in which the body functions. But have they brought us any closer to the achievement of most importance to me, to an understanding of disease itself? I wonder. The more that is revealed, the further the truth recedes. And I am alarmed by the present influence of Descartes's materialism."

The grip on my hand increased and I felt a delicious languor creep through my body. I heard Telesphorus speak as if in a dream.

"My father understood the extent of the suffering you would have

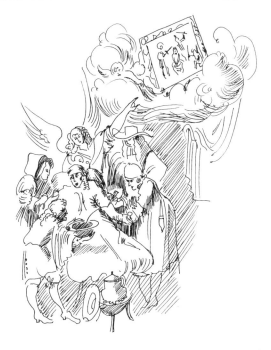

Medicine may have stood at the brink of a great scientific achievement, but the influence of the past was not ready to be shaken off. A blood-letting scene (late seventeenth century) by Romeyn de Hooch (or Hooghe, 1645-1708). In the picture on the wall, one of the Stations of Christ's Passion is demonstrated to the dying man - comparing it, by inference, to the medical scene that is depicted.

to endure and he permitted me, should your mind be close to disintegration, to grant you a glimpse of the future. But you will forget my words as though they were never spoken until the events have taken place; then you will remember with gratitude my telling you.

"Medicine," he spoke as if gathering knowledge directly from another world, "stands at the brink of great scientific advancement. As it moves on, many different paths are to be revealed, so varied and extensive is the knowledge waiting to be acquired. As you – indeed, as any man – will be unable to walk along every one, I shall lead you to those that will increase man's understanding of disease.

"As for Ishtar, I see her returning within a space of time that, compared to the days of your life, is no more than a fleeting moment. Take heart, dear Bal-sarra-uzur."

*   *   *

When I awoke the next day, I felt as though a crushing weight had been lifted from me. I was also not a little surprised to learn that a professor from the university wished to visit me. Accordingly, I sent a messenger with a note to say that, as I was weak from my illness and should not be leaving my house for a while, I should be pleased to receive him at any time.

I have no hesitation in saying that Marcello Malpighi was one of the kindest and most sympathetic of men it had ever been my privilege to meet. The gentleness in his character was evident in every look and gesture, yet there was a touch of sadness in his eye as though he despaired of mankind. He was a modest man – too modest for his own good, was Telesphorus's opinion. Although he suffered from ill-informed criticism, he bore his critics, who in later years included some of his former pupils, no animosity. The reason for the attacks on his studies was due to their being concerned with structures seen through the magnifying lenses of the new-fangled microscope: such detailed scientific knowledge was regarded as useless when compared with the practical knowledge required for the cure of patients – a cry as old as Socrates.

Malpighi held my hand; his grasp was firm while he looked closely at me.

"Yes," he said, "you have indeed been ill and, I would hazard, on the verge of death." Would that I had, and been carried beyond! "But you are restored to health and that pleases me. Might I enquire – as one physician of another – the nature of your sickness?"

I doubt if there was another human being I would have told, but Malpighi inspired confidence; despite this being our first meeting, it seemed I had known him long and intimately.

"I was plunged into a deep melancholia which my assistant and friend, Telesphorus, would have me believe was the insanity of love*. Perhaps he is correct though, as I am recovered, I no longer speak of the circumstances; they are too painful. But why did you wish to see me?"

"Among the many rumours attending your arrival in the city and your known desire not to enter into society, was one that you had come from London. Was that so?"

"Yes."

"And you did speak with the Englishman, William Harvey?"

"That is true."

"Then you know there was one crucial hiatus in his demonstration of the circulation of the blood. Because he saw no connecting channels, he was compelled to postulate the existence of pores in the lungs and tissues to account for the continuous flow from arteries to veins. He *could* not see them. I have seen them!"

His words conveyed the joy of intellectual achievement, not of triumphant boasting. My expression must surely have made him fearful of a return of my insanity.

"You do not believe I can be speaking the truth?" He answered my amazement.

"No! No! I believe you. What I cannot believe is how such a miracle is possible."

"Then you shall accompany me to my laboratory as soon as you are fully recovered and see for yourself."

Suddenly my weakness left me and I was eager to see this wonder without delay. Together we walked to the university.

The preparations for the demonstration were soon completed.

"While the heart is still beating," he was lucid in his description as he bent over my shoulder, pointing to what I should note, "you can see the movements of the blood in the vessels in the opposite directions, so that the fact of its circulation is clearly laid bare. This, you will more

---

* As the diagnosis of mental disease was as much a matter of fanciful speculation as anything else, insanity due to love was extensively written about in the sixteenth (mainly) and seventeenth centuries. – J.G.

readily observe in the mesentery and other larger veins in the abdomen. Thus the blood cascades in minute streams through the arteries into the different cells. The stream repeatedly divides, loses its red colour and, carried round in a sinuous manner, is poured out on all sides until it approaches the walls of the absorbing branches of the veins."

Malpighi stood back. The hedgehog had died.

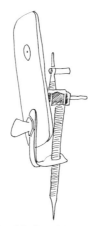

"You have to look to Leeuwenhoek with his beautifully ground lenses if you wish to discover the real creator of the science of microscopy." The small lens was firmly clamped between the two brass plates, while the specimen was mounted on the pointed holder opposite. Focusing was achieved by the use of the screw adjustments which could move the specimen in two directions. One lens was preferred to two, since the use of two would only compound the optical distortions of the lenses, inevitable at this period unless, perhaps, ground by Leeuwenhoek himself. At best, Leeuwenhoek may have achieved a magnification of x 270.

"The eye can see no more in the opened living animal," he said as I turned to face him. "So, you might argue, the blood itself has escaped into an empty space and has been gathered up again by the mouth of a gaping vessel and by the structure of the walls. But I would answer that the movement of the blood is tortuous, scattered in all directions, and is united again at a definite point.

"For this argument to be resolved, you must come over here." He led me to another bench where lay the dried lung of a frog. He handed me a more powerful microscope lens.

"The redness of the blood is preserved to a very great extent in minute tracks, which are vessels joined together in ring-like fashion. Such is the meandering about of these vessels as they proceed from the artery on this side, and to the vein on the other, that they no longer keep to a straight direction. Instead, the continuations of the two vessels appear to make up a network. This network not only occupies the whole area but extends to the walls and is attached to the outgoing vessels – I can show this more abundantly, but with more difficulty in the oblong lung of the tortoise.

"Hence," he went on, greatly pleased at my interest, "hence, it is evident that the blood flows away along tortuous vessels and is not poured into spaces. It is always contained within tubules and its dispersion is due to the multiple winding of the vessels.

"When I made these discoveries, I wrote of them to Borelli. He is a mathematician, you know, and he considers physiology to be a branch of physics. He will be intrigued by some of the other things I have seen. Were you aware that the lungs are not of a muscular consistency? No? They are made up of a multitude of extremely thin-walled compartments which are connected to the final minute filaments of the bronchi. And I have seen fat globules in the blood vessels which resemble nothing so much as rosaries of red coral*."

"Did you invent this instrument yourself?" I was intensely curious about this invention which had turned speculation into reality.

"No. Magnifying lenses have been in use both singly and in combination for some years. You have to look to Leeuwenhoek with his beautifully ground lenses if you wish to discover the real creator of the science of microscopy."

Throughout the years that followed, I maintained a correspondence with Malpighi and his letters contained detailed descriptions, accompanied by the most delicate drawings, of the minutest components of innumerable organs and tissues. The last letter I received was, though, unutterably sad.

"I live," he wrote, "if it can be called life, in idleness without other aim than to distract my grief. A chance fire in my house in the last month has burned what little I had, my manuscript notes, my microscopes and lenses – only one was saved and this, with a small sum of money, was stolen a short time afterwards. I must recognize in

---

* These "fat globules" were rouleaux, a column-like formation that the red blood cells assume under certain conditions. The red cells had, in fact, been discovered six or seven years earlier by the Dutch physician and experimenter (amongst other things, he developed the wax technique of injecting anatomical specimens), Jan Swammerdam (1637 – 1680). – J.G.

this the voice of heaven, the more that to my old ills there are added particular pains which fetter me close so that nothing remains to me but to study and enjoy as best I can the work of others."*

*   *   *

I doubt whether that study would have given him much enjoyment. The advancement of science through the microscope failed to impress the physicians. Indeed, those who dealt with the sick saw little or no profit in any of the wealth of new anatomical and physiological discoveries. They were far more concerned with gaining experience through the exercise of their own observational skills.

"Paolo, I think we should journey to England again." Telesphorus's thoughts about my travels and destinations were less suggestions, more decisions already taken. "I believe you should meet a great exponent of the art of bedside medicine before it is too late. He is, as the English would say, a martyr to the gout and it seems likely to kill him."

And so I found myself once more in Robert Boyle's lodgings in London, alone this time, with one of his closest friends, Thomas Sydenham. It was autumn and his gout was in abeyance. He was a man of pleasing appearance, unassumingly dressed as befitted a one-time soldier who, as a youth, had been a captain in the Parliamentary army during the English Civil War. Hoping to get our conversation off on the right foot, I began by asking which books he would recommend in order to acquire medical knowledge.

"Peruse Don Quixote," was the revealing answer.

He smiled. "Let me explain. I have, myself, been very careful to write nothing but what was the product of faithful observation and neither suffered myself to be deceived by idle speculation, nor have deceived others by obtruding anything upon them but downright matter of fact. And, furthermore, symptoms should be recorded with the same minuteness and accuracy as is observed by a painter painting a portrait."

He went on to show me his writings on a number of diseases. Those I remember best were on gout (which was agonizingly informed from his own experience), the measles, an epidemic cough with fever [this, Dr Annandale, you would recognize to be influenza] and scarlet fever. I was able to read them within the space of a few minutes, so concise

---

* Malpighi wrote a similar letter to his old friend, Francisco Redi (1626 – 1697). Redi was the first man to demonstrate that the popular belief in the spontaneous generation of matter was false. – J.G.

and masterful was his style and containing all that a physician would require to make the diagnosis and prescribe the treatment. They also made plain that, since each patient was a unique human being, the manifestations of a given disease might vary from person to person. He was truly a physician in the direct line from Hippocrates.

I returned the papers. "I am fascinated. You mention the manifest qualities of the air as being responsible for the epidemic cough, and scarlet fever attacking mostly children and at the end of the summer; while gout, when regular, comes on at the end of January or the beginning of February. Your observations would indicate that climate and weather govern some aspects of disease."

"Many things influence the occurrence of disease," Sydenham responded. "As you say, the adequacy and foulness of the air and the seasons mark out the occurrence of many fevers. But health or ill-health depends on much else besides. The physician must heed the sufficiency and quality of what is eaten, the exercise that is taken, also rest and sleep, the calmness or perturbation of the mind, and the state of the bowels and the passing of the urine. All are to be considered by the observant physician."

He fell into a moment's contemplation. Raising his head, he continued:

"But of one thing I can assure you, the stars neither cause diseases nor influence their natural courses. Do not believe those who tell you otherwise!"

"And treatment?" I enquired.

"I generally follow the practice of my fellow physicians, except in two notable respects. I give quinquina or the Jesuits powder for the malarial fevers – though it finds no favour with many. And it is not always necessary to treat with medicines; in many instances I look to my patients' safety and to my own reputation most effectively by doing nothing at all!"

Did I detect a lingering echo of my first master, Imhotep?

16

Symptoms gain anatomical meaning*

alpighi was dead when I returned to Bologna**. He had lived on, plagued by vomiting, bilious stools and kidney stones, for ten unhappy years after the fire. As I received no reply to my letters I had, at length, stopped writing.

With the changing times I was finding it increasingly difficult to keep a home in any one city for too long and I did not take kindly to Telesphorus's subtle alterations to my appearance to create the illusion of increasing age. Sometimes, though, when I returned after a relatively brief span, I could do so as my own son. On these occasions Telesphorus would have retained the property and always, by some miracle, would have both house and garden prepared for my homecoming, unchanged as though they had never been deserted.

I strolled, at ease with myself, in the garden rejoicing in the myriad of scents, cupping a bloom here and there between the fingers of my hand or simply gazing in wonderment at each well-remembered and treasured plant. The tour of inspection completed and old acquaintances renewed, I made my way to the arbour where I settled myself in delicious comfort and let my mind wander.

* The birth of pathology 18th century. – J.G.
** It is ironic, really, considering the content of this part of Paul Baldassare's story, that the details of Malpighi's last illness (he died of a severe stroke) and of the treatment he received, were recorded by his physician, Giorgio Baglivi (1669 – ?1707), together with an account of the post-mortem conducted by Baglivi and Giovanni Maria Lancisi (1654 – 1720) on December 7, 1694. Two pints of clotted blood were found in the cavity of the right ventricle of the brain. "The Blood Vessels of the Brain were dilated and broke on all Hands." – J.G.

My visit to Sydenham had persuaded me that if medicine were finally to shake itself free of the past, the physician had to heed discoveries in anatomy and physiology and adapt them for practical use at the bedside. But this he was unlikely to do until he could grasp their relevance to diagnosis and choice of treatment. In the meantime, he would continue to rely on what the patient – and the patient's friends and relatives – told him; he would feel the pulse, smell and taste the urine and treat the symptomatic manifestations with greatly misplaced enthusiasm. What else could he do when he had no concept of the effects of the disease on the body – on its inner structure and functioning?

Over our evening meal, I discussed these thoughts with Telesphorus. He was not impressed.

"You should have learnt by now that you cannot have ideas foreign to the time you are inhabiting." He spoke kindly despite the implied rebuke. "But insofar as morbid anatomy – which is what you are talking about – is concerned, a start has already been made by the Swiss, Théophile Bonet. When he was physician to the Duc de Longueville he grew so bored he began to fill his time by collecting all the post-mortem records he could find. In the end he gathered some three thousand. But, alas! the published collection* was irredeemably flawed because Bonet had uncritically accepted the opinions of the original authors...." Telesphorus broke off his story as we both burst into gales of laughter at his wit**. When we recovered, I had a niggling feeling of guilt as Bonet had clearly been making a genuine attempt to move medicine forward. Telesphorus merely gave a not entirely convincing display of contrition. Wiping the tears from his eyes, he continued:

"The knowledge was not yet there for Bonet to group the cases adequately, but even so he failed to use his own initiative. Consequently, the book lacks any semblance of order and is no more than a list of little practical worth.

"So." There was something about the tone of his voice that boded ill for me. "So, I want you to return yet again to Padua."

---

* *Sepulchretum, sive anatomia practica ex cadaveribus morbo denatis.* Geneva; Chouët, 1679. A revised edition with new commentaries by J.J. Magnetus was published in 1700 (Lugduni; Cramer and Perachon). The book is commonly known simply as the *Sepulchretum.* – J.G.

** Telesphorus, speaking in French, had been making a play on Bonet's name: "opiner du bonnet" can be translated as "to go along with the opinion of others". – J.G.

I tried to remonstrate that my home in Bologna was one I had come to love more dearly than any for many a year, but Telesphorus was not to be argued with.

*   *   *

The tradition of the Italian school of anatomists was long and influential, and nowhere more so than at Padua. When I met the current professor, I was left in no doubt that Telesphorus had, yet again, been right in bringing me to the city. Giovanni Morgagni had been taught by a previous occupant of the Chair, Antonio Valsalva who, in turn, had been a pupil of Malpighi. Valsalva's chosen pleasure had been to study the correlation between anatomy and physiology and how this might be disturbed in the presence of disease. He had sown the seed that was to germinate in the work of Morgagni.

I came to know Morgagni as well as I did any mortal man, and if I closed my eyes I could for the moment imagine that time had stood still and that I was once again talking with Malpighi. In appearance, the two men resembled each other not at all, but kindness and understanding spoke in the voices of both. Morgagni was an excellent teacher and it was his sympathetic relationship with his students that led, indirectly, to his great achievement.

"I had been in Padua for nearly thirty years before I started writing the letters that were to become my book." This had recently been published* and he was explaining to me how it had come to be written. "The idea took shape while discussing the deficiencies of Bonet's *Sepulchretum* with a student. Whether he suggested that I should improve upon the work or whether I decided that, as the task needed doing, I should do it myself, I can no longer recall – remember I am in my eightieth year and am going back twenty years. But whichever was the case, I undertook to record the circumstances and findings of all my post-mortems from then onwards. For some reason – which again escapes me – we agreed on a total of seventy letters, which were to be returned to me. You, Paolo, now hold in your hands a book that I hope will contribute to the well-being of mankind."

---

* *De sedibus et causis morborum per anatomen indagatis libri quinque.* Venetiis: Remondiniana, 1761. (*The seats and causes of disease investigated by anatomy in five books.*) In the days before medical societies and journals became widespread, it was quite usual to write to colleagues about one's discoveries before publishing them in book form, but not usually over so long a period as Morgagni! – J.G.

I have always had a love of books, not only for the written words they contain, but also for the feel of them. It is a sensation approaching the sensual; it is as if the spirit of the author is made manifest without the need to read the words. One of my deepest regrets has been my inability to build a library of all the books that have passed through my hands. Every collection I have attempted has either been dispersed or destroyed – most frequently the latter.

And now, holding Morgagni's book – or should I say books, as it was in two volumes – I felt I was touching his very soul. I asked leave to sit and turn the pages.

"Indeed, yes, my friend," he said, "but first let me explain how it is arranged. The volumes contain my accounts of nearly six hundred and forty dissections. In addition I have included the patient's symptoms and the mode of their dying, so that with all the details assembled, I have been able to relate the symptoms during life with my findings after death. Mostly I have been able to identify the diseased organ responsible for the symptomatic manifestations.

"You will see that diseases are often represented many times. It is always possible to learn something new and the more frequent the dissections, the more reliable are the conclusions likely to be. As I say to my students: 'Those who have dissected or inspected many bodies, have at least learnt to doubt; while others, who are ignorant of anatomy and do not take the trouble to attend to it, are in no doubt at all.'

"Now, Paolo, I must leave. I have other work to attend to, but you are welcome to stay."

And so I remained in his room for the rest of the day. I was already familiar with some of the cases as he had shown me a number of the letters, but what I was not prepared for was their organized presentation in the book. The five "books" into which the whole was divided were categorized: cerebral disorders; respiratory and cardiac conditions; disorders of digestion and the genito-urinary tract; fevers, tumours, traumatic and surgical conditions; and miscellaneous states together with further deliberations on previous cases. Cross-references abounded and Morgagni never failed to give credit to other writers whose work he cited as adding to the authority of a point he was making.

As I leafed through, I soon noticed there was even more information than he had suggested. He had included personal details about the patients: apart from their age and whether or not they were married, he had recorded the illnesses they had suffered previously, the nature of their occupation and, with Hippocratic percipience, any apparently relevant details about the weather and climate. And, on occasion, he had paid attention to the sicknesses that had affected other members of the family.

The skill with which he had identified the salient features, both in life and in death, was masterful. One case I particularly remember since the impression it left on my memory was of the old order giving way to the new.

An epidemic in Padua one winter had spread "especially in some convents of nuns. In one of them all who had contracted it had died. It was obvious that there was nothing contagious as none attending the sick had contracted the disease and even some who had been most careful to keep away from them had contracted it – but not without a particular cause and disposition in almost every one." Those particular causes had included injury to the chest and "infirmity of the powers of the thorax and lungs, such as occur in those of decrepit age".

"Although three different physicians had attended, not one of the sick could be saved; yet many ascribed the deaths to the unknown nature of the disorder rather than the intensity." [Evidently, Dr Annandale, the cloak of superstition had not been shaken from the people's backs.]

On the death of the tenth patient, a virgin aged forty-two years who every winter had had a violent cough, Morgagni said: "Come let the body be dissected; it is certain to be in the nature of the disease that the lungs shall appear to have the substance of the liver." And so it proved. [From these excerpts, Dr Annandale, you will have no difficulty in recognizing the disease as lobar pneumonia (the old man's friend, as your father would have said) and the origin of the term hepatization to describe the pathological state of the lungs. But Morgagni's full report would, I do not hesitate to say, still bring considerable credit to the physicians and morbid anatomists of your own day.]

As I read on, I realized that now, for the first time, physicians would be able to form a definite picture in their minds of what was happening inside the body. The origin of the symptoms described by the patient would have anatomical meaning which, if interpreted intelligently would help to guide the choice of treatment. In these seventy letters, Morgagni had sounded the death knell of humoral medicine. No longer could it be rationally argued that disease had but one cause (a disorder of the humours with all its variations to suit the circumstances); it was now evident that many different morbid processes could incapacitate or destroy the body.

I felt a sense of great elation.

*　　*　　*

Telesphorus soon brought me down to earth.

"Master, you run too fast," was his response to my account of Morgagni's work. "Despite the title of his book, he has brought the physician no closer to understanding the causes of disease; the causes of the symptoms maybe, but not of disease. Has he brought you closer to your release or merely conceived another possible solution to the insoluble problems of disease and death?"

He saw the look of horror cross my face. "It may be, as I think you realize, that the problem is insoluble only to man, not to the gods."

What was I to make of this? As I understood him, Telesphorus was saying that as ideas about disease changed, man would believe himself closer to the truth. Yet the belief would be merely illusion. To paraphrase Morgagni: in the past man was in no doubt at all, but as his knowledge increased, so did his doubts.

I was relieved when Telesphorus let the subject drop. He knew he had given me much cause for thought.

After Morgagni's death, I returned to my Bologna home as the third generation of the Baldassare family to reside there. Once again, I found the place just as I had left it. But one morning, I forget how many years later, I awoke to a musty smell about the house; the curtains hung awry and would have fallen in shreds had they been drawn. My beautiful furniture looked to have lain for years in a leaking attic. The building itself had decayed and when I stepped into the garden I could not restrain my tears: the paths I had walked along were submerged in undergrowth and none of my chosen flowers would bloom again. The wall around my physic garden had crumbled. My home lay desolate. Telesphorus was nowhere to be seen.

I drew back indoors. The surface of the reception table in the hallway was surprisingly bright and shone in the sunlight; on it lay a brightly polished salver holding a note addressed to Doctor Paul Baldassare.

"It is time to move," the note read. "Nothing remains for you in Italy. Come to Paris."

How typical of Telesphorus! He first plays with time and then commands me without even troubling to sign the note. Nevertheless, I could imagine the twinkle in his eye as he planned a campaign that would both impress me with the passage of time and leave me no choice but to obey. Once this had sunk in, I even found it in my heart to forgive him the destruction of my home. He had, after all, been responsible for the halting of its natural decay and now had simply permitted time to catch up with itself.

*   *   *

When my coach slithered through the January mire into Paris, the Revolution that had torn France apart had long been over and the Republic was now ruled by an executive consisting of a three-man Consulate. The politics of the matter concerned neither Telesphorus nor myself.

"Paul," he said, before I had even had the opportunity to commend him on his choice of a fashionable house on the south bank of the river; from the upper rooms I had an excellent view over the city towards Montmartre in the distance. "I have arranged for you to meet Marie-François-Xavier Bichat – though why the French indulge themselves in these strings of hyphenated names is beyond my comprehension – at the school of anatomy. He has progressed beyond Morgagni."

And so it was that I spent a pleasant morning in the company of Bichat. At once I realized he had an ungovernable urge to bring order to everything and in his latest outburst he had classified the tissues of the body into twenty-one groups. Quite how he managed this, still puzzles me as he disdained the use of a microscope, believing it to be responsible for distortion which could lead to false conclusions.

"If dissection does not give me satisfactory results, I resort to desiccation, maceration, putrefaction and the use of chemical agents."

Although I quickly grasped the reasoning behind these techniques, I could not stop my eyebrows rising in surprise, but he seemed not to notice.

"Medicine has been excluded from the exact sciences for a long time," he continued, "but it will have a right to be associated with them, at least as regards the diagnosis of disease, when we shall have combined clinical observation with the examination of the alterations suffered by the organs in every disease. Of what value is clinical observation if one is ignorant of the seat of the evil?"

I looked questioningly at Telesphorus. "But this is what Morgagni said," I muttered. His glance held the unmistakable message to be silent.

In the next moment my question was answered.

"You are aware, Dr Baldassare, are you not, that my anatomical studies have identified twenty-one different tissues in the body?"

I acknowledged that to be so.

"Morgagni related the clinical symptoms to the organs of the body. I have gone further and related them to the tissues. The more I observe diseases in the opened cadaver – and I have examined more than six hundred – the more am I convinced of the need to consider local disease, not from the point of view of complex organs but from that of the individual tissues.

"It is impossible ever to explore too deeply." His eyes held the look of a visionary. "Dissect in anatomy, experiment in physiology, follow the disease and perform the necropsy in medicine. This is the three-fold path without which there can be no anatomist, no physiologist, no physician."

Telesphorus had summoned me to Paris just in time. Two days after our meeting, Bichat cut himself with his scalpel while dissecting. At the age of thirty-one he became a casualty in the words of Jean-Nicolas Corvisart, "on the field of battle that numbers more than one victim".

17

The proper study of mankind is man*

battlefield of quite a different nature, and one whose casualties down the ages are numbered in their millions, faced Dominique Jean Larrey.

Alexander of Macedon and Napoleon Bonaparte both suffered from the same fatal disease: neither knew when to stop. Alexander stepped beyond the limits set for him by the gods. Napoleon lost his sense of timing – an event that he himself had foreseen. You might say that he, too, was deserted by the gods. But when Telesphorus, evidently growing bored with my academic existence and feeling the need of excitement, drew my attention to an unlikely order signed by the First Consul, that disease had not yet taken hold.

I doubt whether Napoleon – for it was he who was the *First* Consul, let no man think otherwise – fully realized what he was signing when Larrey placed the document before him. It gave Larrey, first surgeon to the Consular Guard and to the Hospital of the Guard, the authority to appoint his own nominees to vacancies in both the Hospital and the surgical service of the Guard. This put the nose of the Administration de la Guerre** quite out of joint.

Strange as it may seem, Napoleon and Larrey had two things in common – strange because one was responsible for the slaughter of

* Casualty evacuation in the Napoleonic Wars. 1802 – 1815. – J.G.
** The reasons for the antagonism between the Administration and both the fighting man and the medical services are lost in the dark recesses of history. But make no mistake, it was very real. – J.G.

millions and the other for clearing up the mess to the best of his very considerable ability. One of these things was an intense irritation with the Administration, a perpetual thorn in Napoleon's flesh and the bane of Larrey's entire career. The other was that both were idolized by the army.

So, at Telesphorus's behest, I took myself to the Hospital of Gros Caillou to begin my fitful career as Surgeon-Major Paul Baldassare of the Guard. At first I wondered what Telesphorus had been thinking about as the French army was on a peacetime footing and Larrey was running a course on experimental surgery at the Val-de-Grâce school of military medicine. However, after I had been Larrey's assistant for a year, the answer came loud and clear: England declared war on France.

The First Consul responded by ordering a period of intensive training for a projected invasion of England. But no sooner was this under way than it ceased to have interest for me. My heart was in a tumult of delight.

Cherubini's *Medée* was being revived at the Paris Opera at the personal request of the First Consul as part of his design to restore the privileged splendour of the past. In the title role was its creator, Julie-Angélique Scio. And, included in the First Consul's suite at the first night, were Larrey, Madame Larrey and myself. At that time I was unfamiliar with opera – with music generally – but I knew my Euripides and was intrigued at the thought of seeing the musical transformation of his play. The Overture set the scene perfectly with its seriousness and intimations of the tragedy that was to come. But I only began to feel my emotions involved when Jason attempted to reassure Glauce, his bride-to-be, that Medée was no threat to their future happiness.

And then Medée, Jason's abandoned love, entered. It was my Ishtar! Fortunately her entrance was greeted with riotous applause, otherwise my intake of breath would have had all eyes turned towards me. In her first impassioned aria I knew she was singing, not to the character with her on the stage, but to me: "You shall never forget your love for me." My emotions were in turmoil when she began to curse Jason for his ingratitude.

How I survived the remainder of that evening, I shall never know. Ishtar/Julie-Angélique was on stage for almost the entire last two acts displaying Medée's passions with such power and dramatic intensity that she could have been Medée incarnate. Her rage as she held the front of the stage while the wedding proceeded behind her was frightening. Cherubini's genius can never have been more in evidence as Medée moved from speech, through accompanied speech to recitative, and to an ungovernable outburst with full orchestra.

The onslaught on my senses right to the final curtain when Medée's vengeance was complete and the knowledge that Ishtar was mine again were more than I could bear. I sat numbed in body and mind until, as the tumult of applause died away, Larrey, a concerned look on his face, shook my arm. Reality of a sort returned; I no longer cared what the First Consul or, indeed, any other human being, might think – my actions were beyond my control. Heedless of the danger from the footlights I leapt onto the stage and, fighting off restraining hands, found my way to Madame Scio's dressing room. She was utterly drained, physically and emotionally, by her performance, but as soon as I burst in she dismissed her dressers and we touched.

Ishtar had returned to me. The soul did indeed become incarnate in another body – or was it in the same body but in a different time?

My home in Paris was in the cul-de-sac Conti at Monnaie and, when Julie-Angélique had recovered sufficiently, we were driven there in her carriage. We had refused the command of the First Consul to attend his celebratory gathering with the excuse of her exhaustion – which alas! was all too close to the truth. We fell asleep before the oil in the lamp had run dry.

"How," I asked the next morning, "did you know you had returned to me?" Studying her in the light of day, I could see images of her previous incarnations, yet there was one I could not recognize – and it was not Julie-Angélique herself. I felt I was seeing Ishtar the priestess in a form that reflected centuries of indefinable change, as if a wheel had turned full circle.

Her answer to my question was simple. "I had not the slightest hint of my previous existences until Etienne – he was my husband – died seven years ago; then I began to have dreams that impressed their message on my innermost being. It was as if I was being prepared for your arrival. I was taught everything that had happened to me, to us. And then last night I sensed you were out there and I sang to you. It was the performance of my life."

And that, too, was the critics' verdict. One wrote that her voice "filled the soul with a kind of astonished wonder, as though it beheld a miracle." And another, "Madame Scio is a divinity among mortals." (He was truer than he could ever have guessed!) "When she throws out her voice to the utmost it has a volume and strength that are quite surprising; while its agility in divisions, running up and down the scale in semitones, is equally astonishing. Hers is a voice of great beauty, remarkably even and admirably disciplined throughout its extensive range." (I am assured by Telesphorus that this was praise indeed!)

But that performance had taken its toll and she was compelled to cancel her next appearance. As the days passed I began to suspect that all was not well with her. But she managed to fulfil her remaining commitments and then, at the season's end we were married.

The following spring the newly-crowned Emperor Napoleon put into operation his plan to lure the English fleet away from the Channel. On his orders, Larrey and I reported to the Imperial headquarters at Bologne where we found the army of invasion already embarked. When the fleet failed to arrive to cover our crossing, the Emperor marched instead into Europe to drive a wedge between the Austrian and Russian armies which were reported to be uniting against him.

The Grande Armée – the name given by the Emperor himself to the new-formed army – had crossed the Rhine before the enemy was even aware of its existence. The march continued swiftly towards the Danube in a great sweep behind the Austrian position. After some skirmishing on the banks of the river, the advance guard forced a crossing at Donauwörth. Here, for the first time, I was in action with Larrey's flying ambulances. These vehicles – two- or four-wheeled, well sprung vehicles with floors that could be slid out to serve as stretchers – lay at the heart of a complete system of casualty evacuation which Larrey had devised towards the end of the wars of the Revolution.

"They can follow the most rapid movements of the advance guard." Larrey had explained their tactical deployment to me. "When necessary, they can separate into a great many subdivisions, since every medical officer is mounted and has at his command a flying ambulance, a mounted orderly, and everything required for giving the earliest assistance on the field of battle.

"The casualties rescued by the flying ambulances," he had continued, "are assembled with all speed at a central point where the surgeon-in-chief or a competent surgeon under his direction, will operate on the most seriously wounded. Always start with the most dangerously injured, without regard to rank or distinction." And with that injunction, Larrey was to tread on many self-important toes.

The Grande Armée marched on through appalling weather, mud at times up to our waists, with Ney having a hard fight to dislodge the Austrians from the abbey at Elchingen. When victory was ours, Larrey had the casualties of both sides collected in what remained of the abbey and we attended them in order of medical priority and, as Larrey had demanded, regardless of nationality. And this, since dressings were in short supply, greatly displeased the French officers.

The Emperor next proceeded to out-manoeuvre a large part of the Austrian army and to force their surrender at Ulm. Then, after some vicious engagements, he took Vienna and marched north-east to confront a combined Austro-Russian army. A major battle was now inevitable and Larrey busied himself making arrangements for the reception of the wounded – among his many talents was his ability to estimate accurately the number of casualties to be expected from a battle. He commandeered the convents and civil hospitals, and – as its Surgeon-in-Chief – reserved the almshouses for the Imperial Guard. Since the Surgeon-in-Chief of the Grande Armée itself, Pierre François Percy, was still in Vienna organizing the hospitals, Larrey was ordered by the Emperor to take overall surgical charge. Having made our inspection, Larrey wrote to the quartermaster at Brünn. He showed me the letter:

"His Majesty has made me responsible for the medical services of the army and, acting on his verbal orders, I pray you to send me tomorrow morning a sufficient number of carriages for the transport of the wounded; meat and brandy for each ambulance; and all the stretchers you have available.

"Will you also instruct the divisional quartermasters to report tomorrow morning to the three main field dressing stations. From there we will be able to dispatch as many subdivisions as will be needed to follow the advancing columns even if they pursue the enemy far and wide.

"Today, I inspected the ambulance divisions and the medical officers of the army corps. I told them where to find instruments and dressings on the field of battle and entrusted their care to the senior surgeons. I shall repeat my inspection tonight.

"I think these measures and my own overall supervision will give

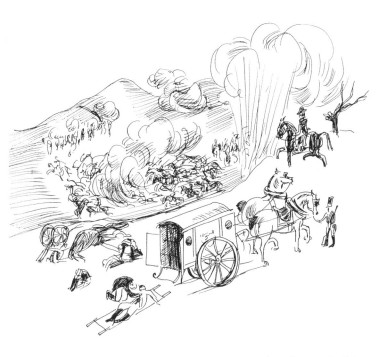

Larrey's flying ambulances lay at the heart of the complete system of casualty evacuation that he had devised. "They can follow the most rapid movements of the advance guard."

the wounded all the help they have a right to expect of us. I only urge you to act most speedily in supplying my needs."

He took the letter back. "Well, what do you think?"

"Only that there will be one furious quartermaster in Brünn when he reads it."

I was right. For a quartermaster to be told what to do by a mere surgeon even though the orders emanated from the Emperor was not to be countenanced!

As darkness descended on December the first, the freezing rain and hail that had made the last day of waiting one of sheer misery, gave way to clear starry skies and the promise of fine weather. Close on one hundred thousand men of the Grande Armée in bivouac on the hillsides forgot their discomfort in an ecstasy of enthusiasm as their Emperor passed through their ranks.

We did not sleep that night. The first hint of what the day was to bring came when the stillness was broken by a distant cannonade. But in their desire to turn the French right (the cause of the gunfire) the allied army had abandoned the key to its position. When the sun broke through the morning mist the commanding heights of Pratzen were bare; the conspicuous bayonets and artillery of the previous day had gone.

Percy arrived early from Vienna so, at the height of the battle – which lasted from six in the morning until eight at night – we were able to give all our attention to the cavalry of the Imperial Guard, a number of whom had been wounded in a furious charge by their Russian opposite number. We carried out all the necessary operations and dressings on the field and then had the casualties taken by flying ambulances to the main field dressing station in the Paleny mill. These vehicles were so speedy that subsequently we were able to use them for evacuating the wounded of the line. We continued working on the field until four the next morning – the items requested of the quartermaster arriving at midnight! Later that day Larrey sent me back to the hospital at Brünn with those of the wounded who were fit enough to travel.

With tragic swiftness after they had reached Brünn, the wounded of the line and the Russian prisoners, crowded into the often-makeshift hospitals, were overwhelmed by an epidemic of camp fever and, to add to their misery, hospital gangrene became rife*. Fortunately, the wounded of the Guard remained virtually free from these diseases, since the almshouses Larrey had reserved for them were remote from the other hospitals and from the populous parts of the town; they were, moreover, well-aired, well lit and kept perfectly clean.

Before leaving, I had given a report to the Emperor on the state of the casualties. When I had finished, he had looked at me with a far-away expression and made what I thought was a most revealing remark:

"One has only a certain time for war. I shall be good for another six years; after that I must stop myself."

The battle was named Austerlitz, after a poor little village nearby.

*　　*　　*

---

* Camp fever was typhus. Hospital gangrene occurred when a wound became infected with virulent bacteria leading to septicaemia and, as often as not, to death. – J.G.

We arrived home in the spring and I could almost believe that fate had ordained it thus. Larrey was greeted with delight by his beloved Laville and I... can I describe my emotions at being reunited with my Julie-Angélique? I went to all her appearances both in opera and on the concert platform. She sang with the voice of an angel. Yet whenever we came home after a performance she was taking an increasingly long time to recover. Moreover, rumour was spreading in Paris that the role of Medée had consumed her. It was true and I knew she was dying. She must have felt the same, for often she appealed to me: "I'm not going to die, am I?" And always I answered: "No."

At what was to prove to be her last public performance – a recital at the Opera – I thought she looked pale and thin standing alone on the stage surrounded by banks of flowers. The programme was of her own choosing and, as if with the gift of prophesy, she opened the second half with "Divinitées du Styx", the aria from Gluck's *Alceste* in which Alceste offers to die in place of her husband.

That night I had to carry her to bed.

"My talent has destroyed me." Her glorious voice would be heard no more. She could scarcely speak as I sat holding her hand on the last awful day. "But our love survives; not even the gods could kill that." I waited for her breathing to recover. "I have to die and I am happy to die with you beside me. Perhaps – one day – we shall die together."

Why did the gods always decree that my adored Ishtar should die before our earthly love had run its course?

*   *   *

And so, until the Grande Armée and the Imperial Guard were no more, I served side-by-side with Larrey in every campaign, continually at odds with the Administration and watching the genius of a great commander crumble into defeat. The whole business of war was becoming too big for him to exercise the control he had done at the outset of his career. If only he had stopped after those six years! The spark was dying and the moral fibre becoming overstretched. Most of his best and most reliable marshals were being killed and too many of his old grognards, his grumblers, who would willingly have followed him into the jaws of hell were doing just that – and not returning.

If it is true that an army is only as good as its medical services, the Emperor was doomed from the moment he launched his campaigns in the year following our withdrawal from Moscow. The quartermasters all but refused to gather the material for our ambulances and had no wish to issue us with the light carriages or the pack horses needed to carry the first-aid dressings. We lacked practically everything. And that was not all. The hospitals from Dresden to the Rhine and beyond were truly called the sepulchres of the Grande Armée. Camp fever swept through the lines of evacuation like an avenging angel.

As Larrey wrote at the close of his campaign journal of that year: "To perform a task as difficult as that which is imposed on a military surgeon, I am convinced that one must often sacrifice oneself, perhaps entirely, to others: must scorn fortune and maintain absolute integrity." In fulfilling this task he did more for mankind than did the Emperor he served so loyally – and received precious little recognition except in the hearts of the common soldier.

[Larrey showed me, Dr Annandale, that even if we may not be able to understand the nature of disease we should, at the very least, try to understand the nature of our patients. As your poet, Alexander Pope, wrote: "Know then thyself, presume not God to scan; / The proper study of mankind is man."]

18

*The stethoscope reveals signs of disease and
its inventor explains their meaning**

he early years of the Second Restoration were hard for
those who had sided with Napoleon – and lacked the
influence or bare-faced effrontery to extricate themselves.
For some, the persecution extended beyond social ostracism to their
work and in Larrey's case the only appointment no one dared take from
him was that of Chief Surgeon of the (now Royal) Guard: his patients
would never have permitted such a liberty.

I had thought to throw in my lot with him, but Telesphorus had
other ideas.

"It will be a long time before others climb on Larrey's shoulders. You
should look to the physicians." And, since he refused to be any more
forthcoming, I could only assume that once again he was surreptitiously
guiding my footsteps. But though I had kept my finger on the pulse of
medical and scientific activities – and they were considerable,
stimulated, as had been so much else, by the fervour of revolution – I
had not the least idea of their destination.

There was one man, though, who might hold the key. I had known
Jean-Nicolas Corvisart reasonably well during the years of the
Consulate and he had always been pleased to discuss medical concerns.
Unfortunately his appointment as personal physician to the Emperor
had produced a rift in our friendship since, jealous of the influence that
Larrey might exert over Napoleon, he had repeatedly thwarted the

* Insturments brought to the aid of diagnosis. 1815 – 1826. – J.G.

surgeon's ambitions at Court – and my sympathies resided firmly in Larrey's camp. I could but hope that Hippocrates's Precept that "healing is a matter of time, but it is also a matter of opportunity" might be applicable out of its original context.

In the intervening years Corvisart had published an important book on the heart* and had translated from the Latin an obscure text on percussion**, neither of which seemed a good enough reason for Telesphorus's injunction. Nevertheless, I decided to seek him out as he was renowned for the excellence of his teaching and for the subsequent brilliance of his pupils. When I had last heard of him he had been Professor of Medicine at the Collège de France and my enquiries revealed that I would still find him there.

He welcomed me as though we had never fallen out – which, in truth, we never had; our friendship had simply cooled. He had changed little; maybe his hair was whiter and the receding hairline was now closer to the back of his head, but his eyes had not lost their kindly quizzical look – a look I have often noticed in the eyes of born teachers. To my consternation, he studied me more closely than I felt was strictly necessary.

"You have worn well," was all he remarked. "Presumably there is a reason you wish to see me again after all this time?" Did I detect a touch of humour in his voice?

"Yes," I answered. I saw no point in dissimulation even though I had concocted what I hoped would seem a compelling reason for my visit. "I have received a letter from a friend in America enquiring about the state of medicine in France now that we are no longer at war. I understand you have developed Morgagni's correlation between symptoms and post-mortem findings by eliciting signs of the disease during life and relating these to the findings after death?"

"I have, and that is why I regard my translation of Auenbrugger's treatise on percussion as of the first importance. His discovery – which

---

* *Essai sur les maladies et les lésions organique du coeur et des gross vaisseaux.* Paris: Migneret, 1806. Corvisart laid emphasis on those symptoms that arose from the heart and helped to clarify the differentiation between cardiac and pulmonary disease. – J.G.
** Auenbrugger L. *Inventum novum ex percussione thoracis humani ut signo abstrusos interni pectoris morbus detegendi.* Vindobonae: Trattner, 1761. Corvisart's translation was published in 1808 as: *Nouvelle méthode pour reconnaître les maladies internes de la poitrine par la percussion de cette cavité, par Auenbrugger.* (See: Oeuvres de Corvisart, vol. II. Paris: Méquignon-Marvis.) – J.G.

was the application of the way he measured the level of wine in his father's casks to what he called hardening of the lungs – has enabled me to estimate during life not only the condition of the lungs, but also the size of the heart. And, what is more, I have confirmed the accuracy of these assessments at post-mortem. Although I am not the first to have translated his book, I am the first to appreciate its merit. In fact, I could have claimed credit for the discovery but, as I wrote in my Preface: 'By that I would sacrifice the name of Auenbrugger to my own vanity and that I do not wish to do: It belongs to him, it is his beautiful and rightful discovery (*Inventum novum*, as he rightly says) which I wish to bring to life.'

"Even so, there is a former student of mine who is pursuing the work of Morgagni, Auenbrugger and myself still further. The correlation of symptoms with post-mortem changes is only the first step in improving our method of diagnosis. It is essential to discover the *signs* of disease so that the picture may be completed. Auenbrugger realized that this was so, but his heart was not truly in his discovery and its disregard by his contemporaries was of small concern to him. Nevertheless, Doctor Baldassare, my translation has attracted attention and as time has moved on, I would recommend you to visit that ex-pupil of mine who is now a physician at the Hôpital Necker."

The next morning was herald to a glorious early autumn day so, looking upon it as a favourable omen, I took a leisurely stroll to the Hôpital. I should have known that René-Théophile-Hyacinth Laennec* always made an early start and consequently he was already well through his rounds. As I arrived he was deep in thought and I contrived to slip unnoticed among the students gathered around the bed. Apparently he was dissatisfied with his examination of a young lady. Percussion and palpation had revealed nothing on account of her fatness, and her age and sex ruled out the use of direct or immediate auscultation. [The ear has been applied directly to the chest wall, Dr Annandale, on and off since Hippocrates described, mainly in culinary terms, some of the sounds he heard; but he did correctly identify the presence of dry pleurisy by likening the sound it produced to that of creaking leather. Difficult though it may be for you to appreciate, the

---

* Laennec did not use the diaeresis (Laënnec) commonly found in the spelling of his name which, nevertheless, should be pronounced in three syllables, not two. – J.G.

concept of structural pathology scarcely existed before the eighteenth-nineteenth centuries and if any physician before then had even bothered to elicit evidence of structural changes within the body, it would have been a complete waste of time as he would have had no idea of its significance!]

Slowly Laennec turned to face his students. I cannot say I was shocked by his appearance, but I could not prevent a silent gasp. He had the look of a man who knew his time was limited. Already the signs of the disease, pulmonary tuberculosis, the nature of which he was to elucidate, were apparent.

"Why," he said after a preliminary cough, "should we not make use of a well-known fact in acoustics? I refer, of course, to the speaking trumpet which enables the hard-of-hearing to be aware of the faintest whisper; to the ascending tube in the warehouse which conveys to the upper storeys the muttered directions of the master below; to the ticking of a watch placed at the end of a long beam or the scratching of a pin which is heard loudly by the ear applied to its other end. Therefore, if I place a tube on the chest over the lungs or the heart I ought to hear the sounds of the movements within more plainly."

And, without further ado, he snatched the notes from the hands of the nearest student and, rolling the papers lengthways, applied one end to his ear and the other, first to one side of the patient's chest, then to the other, and then to her back between and below the shoulder blades.

He raised his head and handed the still-rolled pages back to their owner. His elation was evident.

"I can hear the movements of respiration and the actions of the heart much more clearly and more distinctly than ever I could by the direct application of my ear to the chest." He paused for a moment, contemplating the significance of what he had heard. His drawn face lit up. "I believe we have here the means for enabling us to discover the character, not only of the heart's action, but also the manner of sound produced by every movement of the lungs: we can now explore the nature of respiration!"

As I left the ward, intending to return later in the day, I wondered whether Laennec was the physician Telesphorus had in mind. I decided to call on Larrey on my way home; he might be able to judge the importance of Laennec's discovery.

Before I could speak, he hurried me through the door.

"Baldassare, your name is on the black list and it is only a matter of time before you will be arrested. I hear you insulted a returned royalist emigré. Is that true?"

"And with justification!" I replied with considerable vehemence. "M Carlin, a pompous idiot if ever I saw one, was holding forth on the military incompetence of the 'Corsican upstart'. I simply stared at him. 'The Emperor was worth a hundred of your Bourbon kings, as you would know if you had fought with him for the glory of France,' I said, and turned on my heel."

"Then you certainly must flee Paris, even France; stay away until I write that it is safe for you to return – passions may take a few years to cool. Your services to France cannot save you from the consequences of a treasonable remark like that. Go to England while you are still at liberty."

With that advice ringing in my ears, I escaped to the country that had thwarted the Napoleonic ambition at every turn. Here, Telesphorus and I decided to rest after the rigours of the recent war. I have often asked myself who was to blame for that conflict? Napoleon or the European monarchs lined up, sometimes with him, sometimes against? Was it six of one and half-a-dozen of the other? But then I was not an unbiased witness. Had I not spent those past years serving with the greatest Imperial Guard in history whose Surgeon-in-Chief had been in no small measure responsible for its high morale?

In the same way that the English were making a rite of passage of the Grand Tour of Europe, so we made our own Grand Tour of the British Isles. In the course of this I learnt that Laennec had published his book on mediate auscultation*, as he called his new technique of examination. The stethoscope, the name he gave to his instrument, was at first simply a wooden version of the student's rolled-up notes.

Larrey's letters eventually caught up with me and, to my dismay, he wrote that Laennec's treatise had failed to attract critical acclaim in France. Before long, however, copies of the book – and, just as important, of his stethoscope – began to reach England where their arrival was greeted with far greater enthusiasm. One review concluded: "To the enlightened author, of whom France may well be proud, the

---

* De l'auscultation médiate ou traité du diagnostic des maladies des poumons et du coeur, fondé principalement sur ce nouveau moyen d'exploration. Paris: Brosson et Chaudé, 1819. – J.G.

thanks of Europe are due."

To my regret, I was unable to obtain a copy of the book until, a few years later, I was pursuing an interest in cathedral architecture and found myself in Chichester in the County of Sussex. This city boasted a well-known practitioner, by name John Forbes, and, for what seemed no very good reason, I thought I would pay him a visit. My intuition was rewarded: Forbes had recently completed a translation of Laennec's book* and was only too delighted to talk about *his* book to a fellow physician who had attended one of Laennec's rounds and whom he assumed to be French.

I cannot say that I warmed towards Dr Forbes; he was too sure of himself and regarded his "translation" as an improvement on the original – as, indeed, did some English reviewers! For all his enthusiasm for the sounds – which he comprehensively revised for the benefit of the English reader – he had doubts whether the stethoscope would gain popular appeal.

"Notwithstanding the instrument's value, I confess that the sight of a grave physician solemnly listening through a long wooden tube to a patient's chest has about it an element of the ludicrous." The arrogance of the inhabitants of these Isles amazed me as he continued: "Besides, the method would seem to make a bold claim and to have a pretension to certainty and precision of diagnosis which cannot, at first sight, but be startling to a mind deeply versed in the knowledge and uncertainty of our art, and to the calm and cautious habits of philosophizing to which the English physician is accustomed." I held my tongue: I would have to wait until I could talk to Laennec himself before passing judgment on the matter of diagnostic certainty.

But Forbes continued talking; once launched on his own opinions there was no stopping him.

"Here," he said, his Scottish burr growing more and more irritating to my ears the longer he went on. He was rummaging about in his desk. "No, I cannot find it. I thought I had a copy of the letter I sent to Laennec. Still, no matter, I am reminded of its gist.

"I referred to my book as an abridgement, rather than a translation, of his immortal work. But it was, in fact, more than that. I took

---

* *Treatise on the diseases of the chest in which they are described according to their anatomical characters and their diagnosis established on a new procedure by means of acoustic instruments.* Translated from the French of R.T.H.Laennec, M.D. London: Underwood, 1821 – J.G.

considerable liberties with the manner and matter of his treatise, for which the only substantial excuse I could offer was my conviction that a simple translation of so voluminous a work – I restrained myself from calling its style diffuse and verbose and by no means commendable in a scientific text. As I say, a simple translation would have met with little or no encouragement in this country and would therefore have frustrated the great and important object of making his immortal labours and discoveries known to a large number of British physicians."

I was glad to make my escape from Forbes's home. While he had been talking I had taken the opportunity to leaf through both books. He had, indeed, taken so many liberties that to refer to his "abridgement" as a translation, as he did on his title page, was nothing short of sacrilege. I was now more impatient than ever for Larrey to write assuring me of a safe return to France.

[You may think, Dr Annandale, that I have been unduly harsh on Sir John Forbes considering that it was largely due to his "translations" (which went through several revised editions – changing his choice of descriptive terms as the spirit moved him) that the English-speaking world came to know of Laennec's work on auscultation and his approach to diseases of the chest. But I would be prepared to argue that generations of long-suffering British medical students would have been better served and less confused had Laennec's own terminology for the breath sounds remained untranslated. After all, how many foreign terms are already part of the medical vocabulary? I merely quote from a popular student textbook of not so long ago: "Confusion has been caused by the different terminology employed in different schools." This confusion is far less significant than it used to be, now that the stethoscope is scarcely more than a screening instrument (except to the ears of the expert) before passing the patient on to the x-ray and other more exotic departments. To add to my disgust, all the excerpts in English I have come across of Laennec's writings have been in the Forbes "translation". If you will permit me a final comment on Forbes: he was also responsible for an English translation of Auenbrugger's treatise on auscultation in which he paid scant regard to the subtleties of meanings of many of the terms*.]

*   *   *

* *Original cases with dissections and observations illustrating the use of the stethoscope and percussion in the diagnosis of diseases of the chest; and also commentaries on the same subjects selected and translated from Auenbrugger, Corvisart, Laennec and others.* London: Underwood, 1824. – J.G.

If I had been distressed before at Laennec's appearance, I was truly horrified now, eight years later. His face, never full, had fallen away until the skin was stretched tight over the bone. A hectic flush, combined with the determination in his bright blue eyes, gave him the look of a man not of this world. He had but a short time to live and he knew it – he had seen so many of his patients tread the same path before him. Yet he had so much to do, not the least of which was the completion of the second edition of his *De l'auscultation médiate**.

[Dr Annandale, your English poet and erstwhile surgeon, John Keats knew *The terror of death* from the self-same disease. The opening lines of his poem of that name express Laennec's feelings all too well: When I have fears that I may cease to be / Before my pen has glean'd my teeming brain, / Before high-piléd books, in charact'ry / Hold like rich garners the full-ripen'd grain;...]

"The first edition appeared only three years after I had discovered the use of the baton," he was eager to talk about his work, not self-centredly as was Forbes, but informatively and constructively. "In that time, besides studying, describing and categorizing the sounds, I experimented with the instrument, using different materials and different lengths. I now use a wooden cylinder, an inch-and-a-half in diameter, and a foot long, perforated longitudinally and hollowed out to a funnel shape to a depth of one inch-and-a-half at one of its ends. It can be dismantled into two halves, partly for the convenience of carriage and partly to permit its being used at half its length.

"Although I usually speak of it as a baton or cylinder, I have named it the stethoscope – from the Greek. The precise dimensions are unimportant although I find the full length generally more convenient except when the patient is seated on a chair or in bed, when access is restricted." He was speaking rapidly and with that sense of urgency commonly encountered among those in the final grip of phthisis.

"But my life's work really began long before the arrival of my baton. I was a student of Corvisart at La Charité. He became more of a friend than a teacher and helped me greatly in my career. During the last few years of my formal medical training I prepared, under his supervision, more than four hundred case histories of patients from bedside to post-mortem. So, when I was appointed to the Necker, I had my students

* Published in 1826. – J.G.

keep meticulous notes of the patients in their charge – notes which I supplemented with my own observations; these I dictated in Latin for reasons you will readily appreciate.

"My work at La Charité gave me an excellent grounding in the structural pathology of disease but, so far as the chest was concerned, it lacked the evidence provided during life by the baton..."

Without warning, he broke off in a fit of terrible coughing which nearly broke my heart to hear. When he had recovered, I offered to leave but he insisted on putting straight the matter of Forbes's translation – a copy of which lay open on the desk in front of him – and his charge about the claim made for auscultation.

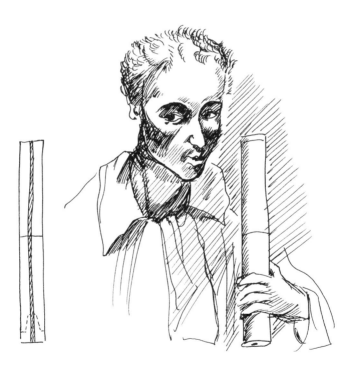

Laennec's appearance was truly horrifying, but he was eager to talk about his work and his invention, the stethoscope. "I now use a wooden cylinder, an inch-and-a-half in diameter, and a foot long, perforated longitudinally and hollowed out to a funnel shape to a depth of one inch-and-a-half at one of its ends. It can be dismantled into two halves."

"M Forbes would never have written those words in his Preface had he spent the three years between discovery and publication here with me at the Necker. Every day I worked to the point of exhaustion. My chief difficulty lay in describing and naming the different sounds I heard – never for one moment did I imagine a greater problem would arise over their translation. But gradually I was able to differentiate them and then to relate them to the pathology revealed at post-mortem. Should the post-mortem show any error in my interpretation, this was corrected immediately in the notes. At first, the sounds I heard merely indicated the nature of the underlying physical state – as you would expect. Then, as I gathered more and more evidence, I believed it safe to say that certain combinations of sounds and physical findings indicated the presence of certain diseases.

"Yes! In that sense, I am guilty of making the claims M Forbes suggests that I do, but they are based on sure evidence, as he would appreciate if he had taken the trouble to examine a sufficient number of patients rather than criticize the work of one who has!"

Laennec's calmness appeared in danger of evaporating. He remained silent for a minute or two and then indicated his readiness to continue.

"The matter of râles and rhonchi?" I queried.

"Ah!" he said, "now you come up against the obtuseness of the English." The ghost of a smile crossed his death-like features.

"In my book, I use the word râles," (when said by Laennec, the word had the hint of an onomatopoeic quality about it, which had been nowhere apparent in the sound produced by Forbes) "indeed, I only use the word in writing. I would never say it in front of a patient as he would associate it with râles de la mort – the death rattle. In England that is not a consideration. So, when speaking to students in front of a patient and dictating my notes in Latin, as I do, I speak of rhonchi, the Latin translation of rattle. M Forbes evidently is ignorant of this fact and believes râles and rhonchi to be two different sounds – no doubt influenced by the homophony of the words rhonchi and bronchi!

"Surely no one could have any problem with my description of the types of râles – or even wish to make a translation!" That ghostly smile appeared again. I liked Laennec. "Râle humide ou crépitation; râle muqueux ou gargouillement; râle sec sonore ou ronflement; râle sibilant ou sifflement. I am now adding a fifth: râle crépitant sec à grosse bulles ou craquement; this is uncommon and I was initially unsure about it which is why I did not include it in the first edition.

"These various sounds occur when there are changes in the underlying lung. The râle sonore when there are changes in the shape or size of the medium or large bronchi – maybe compressed by tumourous growths, lymph nodes or inflammation. If the smallest bronchi are obstructed, the sound is different – more like a prolonged whistle – the râle sibilant.

"Or they may depend on what the air is passing through in the air passages; this may be mucus or tuberculous matter, for example – the râle muqueux; when I hear this in the trachea I imagine the sound is like the wheels of a carriage coming over the paved road to collect the dying patient. Often you can hear it quite plainly without a baton. The râle crépitant sec à grosse bulles is heard only during inspiration and is a crackling sound like the blowing up of a dried bladder; but, as I say, it is uncommon. The râle humide ou crépitation – and here I stand guilty of the charge laid by M Forbes – is the sound I find typical of pneumonia; I can reproduce it in the post-mortem room by gently squeezing the blood-and-air-filled lung.

"I also described most carefully changes in the sound of the voice in disease. The presence of a cavity is indicated by what I term pectoriloquy and I am quite confident that aegophony is heard in cases of pleurisy attended by a moderate effusion or in hydrothorax or other liquid effusion into that cavity.*

"Now, M Baldassare, you shall come with me and listen for yourself to all these sounds and tell me whether an educated physician would require a translation."

I followed him into the ward where he led me from patient to patient, to listen while he told me what I should be hearing, often likening the sounds to the songs of the birds in his beloved Brittany. Had I not had my ear "tuned" by my beloved Julie-Angélique, I swear I would never have recognized the different râles; as it was, I found it remarkably easy to picture in my mind the events within the lungs.

As I was about to leave, he detained me a moment longer.

"Some people think my *De l'auscultation médiate* deals only with my

---

* Although Laennec discovered a cavity at post-mortem in all twenty patients in whom he had encountered pectoriloquy, we now know it can be heard in other states in which there is no cavity. Aegophony is not unlike the bleating of a wild goat (hence the name); the voice sounds have a peculiar wavering tone. – J.G.

stethoscopic discoveries. This is far from being so, though it might appear so to the casual reader of the first edition, since I adopted the analytical approach relating the signs in life to structural pathological changes at post-mortem. In my new edition, however, I have changed that to detailed descriptions of each disease, systematically working my way through diagnosis, pathology and treatment."*

*   *   *

I stood at Laennec's bedside. He was in the act of stepping into the ferryman's boat when he paused, removed the rings from his fingers and laid them gently on the table at his side.

"Because someone would have to render me this service, I wish to spare them the painful task."

I waited until he had arrived safely on the far bank.

---

*This edition has been described as the most important treatise on diseases of the thoracic organs ever written. – J.G.

19

The invisible causes of infection
are made visible*

The medical world – indeed, the world at large – was undergoing cataclysmic change – and I do not exaggerate. The years were gone when Telesphorus and I could wander leisurely from country to country, from town to town, enjoying the talk and experiences of men who were shaping the destiny of medicine. Now the tempo was fast increasing and the very devil of it was that I could not keep pace. But – and this I found infinitely more disturbing – I had an inexplicable sensation that as medicine became more complex, so the prospect of an understanding of disease was receding ever further. [Just like the expanding universe, Dr Annandale!] Had everything I had hoped for been damned from the start?

This troublesome possibility had been sharpened by Ishtar's last manifestation as Julie-Angélique when I had had a strange awareness that there was something different about her; that a wheel had turned full circle. Could it be that she had completed her defined existences on earth, while I was condemned to wait upon events beyond my control? Or, I wondered in my more optimistic moods, could it be that light was there, awaiting its moment to illuminate this medical complexity, to guide mankind to a true understanding? Could it be that my final union with Ishtar was but a few short years away? Unfortunately, the one really unknown quantity in the equation was,

* The start of modern medicine: the contributions of Pasteur and Koch. Mid-19th century – 1881. – J.G.

inevitably, man himself. In consequence, I truly could not define the most important of the many directions medicine was pursuing. Telesphorus, as always, came to my rescue.

"Bal-sarra-uzur, I cannot, to my sorrow, disclose the future to you – my father would banish me from your mortal world for ever should I be so presumptuous and then how could I comfort and advise you? Besides it would remove much of the excitement from life, from both our lives!" It certainly would from his; I was not so sure about mine.

"Come back with me to our old friend Aristotle. You did not know, did you, that he and I spent many mutually enjoyable hours in his belvedere discussing highly abstruse aspects of science and philosophy – I didn't waste all my time in the gynaeceum as you probably believed! Our conversation frequently came up against the nature of life and the topic on one occasion was, as I recall, the various methods of reproduction in the animal kingdom and he was quite adamant that spontaneous generation was a fact of life. This idea of his persisted and for centuries people believed that verminous creatures with no evident means of reproduction originated spontaneously from dung heaps, decaying flesh and vegetable matter and similar obnoxious masses."

"I know Aristotle's teachings have had a profound influence on scientific thinking," I interrupted, "but what in the name of your father has spontaneous generation to do with medicine today when diseases are being unravelled by men such as poor Laennec?"

"Patience, Master, patience. Allow me to pursue the story in my own way and you will see where it leads. But first, as you mentioned his name, what did Laennec believe to be the cause of tuberculosis?"

Telesphorus had caught me unawares.

"I cannot say. But I suppose he subscribed to the popular opinion that it was hereditary, since both his mother and his brother died from phthisis."

"Precisely!" He was triumphant.

I gave him a puzzled look and was about to open my mouth. He raised his hand to stop me.

"Please, Bal-sarra-uzur, I am trying to help you." There was actually a note of pleading in his voice. "For many centuries, spontaneous generation has been accepted as the cause of verminous infestation and decomposition. You have to admit it is a highly plausible explanation."

I refused to comment as I still failed to understand the relevance of his argument to my present predicament.

"An old friend of Malpighi's, Francesco Redi, opened the first crack in the belief." Telesphorus was not to be put off by my obtuse silence. Instead he adopted what I always regard as his professorial voice. "He showed that maggots would appear on meat in uncovered jars, whereas in other jars covered with wire gauze, they still appeared but on top of the gauze. This proved, for those prepared to listen, that it was not the rotting meat that spontaneously produced the larvae (or maggots) of flies; it was simply that the larvae were able to grow on the rotting meat.

"Then Leeuwenhoek put the fly in the ointment." Telesphorus could not contain his merriment and with tears streaming down his cherubic cheeks he nearly slid from his chair. So much for the professor!

When he had gathered himself, he continued: "You remember Malpighi telling you about the Dutchman's exquisite lenses? Yes? Good. Well, with these lenses Leeuwenhoek was able to describe, in detail, the yeast cell. He also reported his observations of minute structures, some of which were in formations like clumps or chains while others were motile. He believed that these 'animalcules', as he called them, came from the air, but his discovery did not, as you might have expected, help towards disproving spontaneous generation, it only made things worse. If, indeed, they did in fact exist outside Leeuwenhoek's imagination, how, people asked, could animalcules come into existence other than by spontaneous generation?

"Other experimenters – I won't bother with their names; you probably wouldn't remember those you had met, anyway – proved, mostly only to their own satisfaction, that spontaneous generation from dead organic matter did not occur. In their different experiments, air was excluded (with varying degrees of success): air was allowed free access. Experiments in which air was heated or passed through acid were condemned on the ground that the air had been deprived of its 'life force' and so animalcules could not be expected to develop.

"I'm sorry, Master, to regurgitate the past like this, but important discoveries rarely, if ever, come unheralded.

"Now, so far as you need be concerned, we are up to date, and what I cannot impress upon you too strongly is that the up-to-date science – and all the metaphors that go with it – is chemistry. Just as the metaphors of Descartes's day were mechanical." The professor was firmly in his chair again.

I thought, nevertheless, it was about time I made an intelligent, if only small, contribution.

"So, as I see it," I said, "there are two conflicting theories, with eminent chemists and scientists proposing convincing and sustainable arguments for both sides. In essence, disease may be caused by animalcules of one sort or another which, according to one theory, are generated spontaneously from organic matter and, according to the other are living organisms, or germs, from the start; they reproduce. Am I correct?"

To my relief and gratification, Telesphorus nodded. "I think you have grasped the essentials of the problem." He could be remarkably condescending when he set his mind to it! "At the present time, the climate of opinion favours the germ theory, though those who contest it have a powerful religious precedent on their side. Spontaneous generation is agreed by many to have occurred 'In the beginning'. So for true believers, it is inconceivable that the process cannot be repeated.

"The real problem confronting the upholders of the germ theory – and I risk incurring the wrath of my father in saying this – is that they have not the slightest idea of how they should study their germs. A theory remains a theory until it receives practical confirmation!"

"Obscurity flourishes in the realm of the invisible." After my intellectual battering by Telesphorus, I felt that was not a bad epigram.

"Quite correct," said the professor in a tone that only just avoided the patronizing. "The number of extremely peculiar ideas circulating among those who cannot accept that germs are able to reproduce themselves is beyond reasonable count. They say that the 'globules' Leeuwenhoek had seen were a form of chemical. They say that 'particles' of an unspecified nature catalyse the normal human chemistry to produce chemical poisons which then cause disease. Other 'particles' have actually been 'proved' experimentally to be the cause of infectious disease. They have been identified as 'spheroidal, transparent, of gelatinous consistence, of density nearly equal to that of the animal liquids in which they float, and that they are mainly, but perhaps not exclusively composed of albuminous matter.' Someone has even claimed he could isolate the poison of hospital fever in solid form! They argue that the growth of crystals in solutions is analogous to the origin of life! Oh, the infinite capacity of man for self-delusion!"

Professor Telesphorus threw up his hands in despair.

Then a thought occurred to him. "Perhaps you are like all the others and are merely a child of the times – as, indeed, you would be if I didn't take you in hand once in a while – and agree with the chemists? The line between the living and the not-living is, in truth, finely drawn.

"Tell me this, Doctor, is yeast a living organism or not? After all, fermentation occupies an important place in our existence." And he took a long draught from the tankard of beer on the table in front of him. "Some chemists regard yeast as a decomposition product of malt and not the cause of fermentation. Have you an opinion on the matter, Dr Baldassare?"

I was silent for a while, thinking furiously. The chemists did seem to occupy the more favourable position. Then a thought occurred to me.

"Telesphorus, answer me this. We are now living in a time when scientific principles are paramount? You agree?" He did. "So theoretical considerations – which constitute most, if not all, the arguments on both sides – must be resolved by enquiries into the conditions under which these lowly organisms, if they exist, can develop and multiply."

"In that case we must visit the Professor of Geology and Chemistry at the Ecole des Beaux-Arts."

As we entered the laboratory, a fine-looking man in his mid-forties stood leaning against a work-bench gazing intently at a sealed flask in his right hand. He acknowledged our arrival with a nod before holding up the flask in our direction.

"I have kept this flask of boiled milk sealed for some time," Louis Pasteur began, a look of controlled excitement taking over from the serious set of his features. "And I wait, I watch, I question it, begging it to recommence for me the beauteous spectacle of the first creation."

Oh, my gods! Telesphorus cannot have brought me to a latter-day alchemist's laboratory; to a reincarnation of Trithemius! Was this one of his little jokes? Was this otherwise intelligent-seeming chemist about to reveal yet another "truth" of spontaneous generation? Yet you do not become a professor at a leading Paris Institute without a certain degree of intellectual integrity.

"But," Pasteur proceeded, "it is dumb, dumb since these experiments were begun several years ago; it is dumb because I have kept from it the only thing Man cannot produce – I have kept from it the germs

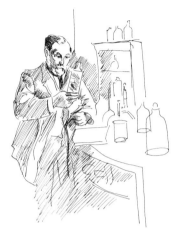

No Trithemius, this man! Louis Pasteur in his laboratory.

that float in the air; I have kept from it Life, for Life is a germ and a germ is Life!"

I sat down, uninvited, on a stool and stared at him.

"I have established," he was in earnest again. No matter how melodramatic his speech, there was nothing of the fanatic about him. "I have established," he said, "that yeast is a living organism and is responsible for fermentation. I have heated wine to fifty or sixty degrees centigrade – which affects neither bouquet nor taste – thus destroying the microscopic organisms that so nearly brought the industry to its knees through spoilage. Since I have proved the utter fallacy of spontaneous generation, I believe that not only have I discovered the causes of fermentation and spoilage, but I have also found the source of life itself!"

He put the flask down on the bench in the one available place between his books, his microscope and his equipment.

"You make no challenge?" He seemed surprised.

"No, since I have no reason," I responded with an encouraging smile.

"You are a strange man, Dr Baldassare." We had been announced by Pasteur's assistant. "Many so-called scientists would have raised trivial objections and continued with their argument that the microscopic organisms I found were produced by spoilage of the wine. Some years ago Thedor Schwann showed yeast to be a living organism but he could not prove that it was responsible for fermentation. The technical difficulties were too many at the time, but time and techniques have moved on and I have been able to resolve the problems."

*   *   *

Pasteur had discovered bacteria* and was putting the information he had gleaned to good practical use. Besides his work for the wine industry, he had been called upon to save the silkworm industry of France which was being crippled by disease. For five years he laboured and when eventually he discovered its cause and how to prevent the disease, his triumph was shattered: "Il y a deux maladies!" Pasteur's cry of despair was echoed by the industry. After more hard, infinitely painstaking work this second disease was also conquered.

Four years after our first meeting, Pasteur suffered a stroke brought on, his friends believed, by the harsh criticism he had had to endure on account of his "failures". I visited him frequently when I was in Paris, as we had developed a sympathetic rapport – he persisted in calling me "you strange man", an indication, if such were needed, that his seriousness did not exclude, only hid, a genuinely warm character. Or did he, like so many intuitive men I had encountered, suspect that I was not what I seemed, yet could not say in what way or give a reason for their suspicions?

Meanwhile the controversy over spontaneous generation rumbled on. I asked Telesphorus why this had not been finally silenced by Pasteur's discoveries.

"It appears you listen neither to yourself nor to me." I feared I was about to be taken to task for a lapsus memoriae, though what particular snatch of conversation I had forgotten was a mystery, but one soon, no doubt, to be uncovered.

"When we were originally discussing the germ theory...."

"But that was twelve years ago." I was indignant. "I am only mortal with a mortal's memory."

"... you yourself said," he ignored my outburst, "that the theoretical arguments must be settled by enquiries into the conditions under which the micro-organisms develop and multiply. A remark obviously inspired by my having said previously that the supporters of the germ theory had not the slightest idea of how they should study their germs! Now

---

* From the Greek, *bakterion*, the diminutive of *baktron*, a stick. – J.G.

argue your way out of that!"

And so I did, very rapidly indeed. "Ah, my dear Telesphorus, you were looking into your crystal ball so, to protect you from the wrath of your father, the words were erased from my memory as soon as they had served their purpose. Now, let us drink to each other and to Louis Pasteur who has again saved from bacterial disaster yet another of mankind's solaces."

We touched beer mugs and muttering "Pasteur, Paul, Telesphorus" (except that Telesphorus spoke his name before mine – the gods do not surrender to mortals that easily), we drank to the last drop.

*　　*　　*

My fear that I might have so upset Telesphorus that it would be a long time before he would proffer even the most obscure of advice, proved quite unfounded – as I should have known it would. It was his suggestion that we should visit Prussia, specifically the region around Breslau*. He would say no more and would give me no reason.

As my clever curly-headed little professor had so amply demonstrated with his sermon on spontaneous generation, I could not keep up with all that was going on in medicine and, on our journey, he proved it once again.

"Dr Baldassare." I knew a lecture was about to be delivered. "Jakob Henle, now Professor of Anatomy at Göttingen, is an exceptionally talented and far-sighted man. His work on microscopic anatomy has carried Bichat's studies onward to include the developmental and functional aspects of the tissues, and his approach to gross anatomy has made it much simpler for students to understand. He is a charming man and possesses great artistic talent – it is a pity you never met him. His lectures are almost lessons in anatomical art; in consequence, his students leave his courses both knowledgeable and inspired.

"One of those students, however, was inspired by something quite other than Henle's anatomy classes. Early in his career, Henle had been fascinated by the problem of contagion and, having accepted that it was due to living micro-organisms, he drew up a set of conditions that had to be fulfilled before a causal association could be established between the suspect micro-organism and the disease in question: The

---

* At the time of their visit, about 1878, Breslau was in Prussia. In 1945 Silesia was annexed by Poland and Breslau was renamed Wrocław. – J.G.

organism had to be demonstrated in every case of the disease and in no other disease. The organism had to be isolated from all other micro-organisms and other extraneous matter. The isolated organism had to be shown to be capable of causing the original disease. Quite demanding criteria, don't you think? Is it any wonder that they were quietly left to simmer until someone found out how bacteria could be studied?

"It has taken a long while for Henle's inspiration to stir the student into action – and it has happened in the most unusual circumstances. Robert Koch, the ex-student, returned from service in the Franco-Prussian War to become district physician at the small town of Wollstein*. He soon grew bored with the monotony of the job and began playing around with his microscope. Before long he realized where his interests and future lay.

"I may have misled you, Balthasar, in saying we were going to Breslau. That is so, but it is not our final destination as I would like you first to meet Julius Cohn. As well as being the Professor of Botany, he is also an enthusiastic bacteriologist; he has already presented evidence that bacteria are constant in their form and has suggested that this could be used as a method of classifying them into genera and species."

But to Telesphorus's annoyance, Professor Cohn was away in Berlin – even the gods can sometimes nod! So on we went to Wollstein.

Koch received us in a fashion that made me feel he would rather be pursuing his studies than entertaining two apparently casual passers-by. Nevertheless, he made us welcome and once I had asked the right question, he agreed to give us a practical demonstration.

For the rest of the day we watched enthralled as he worked through his bacteriological techniques. After staining the fixed preparation with one of the aniline dyes – he used methyl violet, fuchsine or aniline brown, depending on the organism – he examined the slide under the microscope, moving from low power, to high power and then to the oil immersion lens which was quite a new-fangled idea and gave remarkable definition. Finally, he took photographs of the stained bacteria. [Staining the invisible to make it visible, you might say, Dr Annandale.]

"I owe so much to my friend, as he has become, Julius Cohn," he said. "When my first studies – they were on the life-cycle of the bacillus of anthrax – were complete, I wrote to him. He immediately invited

---

* This formerly Prussian town is also now in Poland and goes under the name of Wolsztyn. – J.G.

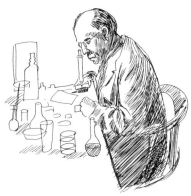

A far cry from Leeuwenhoek. Robert Koch at his home in the small town of Wollstein.

me to demonstrate my methods of culture and staining at his Institute before some of his eminent colleagues. It was a great success.* Soon afterwards, I proved conclusively that micro-organisms were the cause of wound infections. Although this gave the answer to a highly contentious issue, it also gave surgeons much to think about!"

The next time I met Koch – who, by then, was on the staff of the Imperial Health Department – was two or three years later at a medical congress in London where he demonstrated a novel method of obtaining pure cultures on a solid coagulum produced by spreading liquid gelatine and meat infusion on a glass dish.

I had, with difficulty, persuaded Pasteur who had an antipathy to all things Prussian – he had returned his Bonn M.D. at the outbreak of the Franco-Prussian War – to attend the demonstration. Patriot he may have been, but he was even more a great scientist: "C'est un grand progrès!" he exclaimed.

A great progress, it was, indeed. Mankind had at last begun to understand the cause of the array of diseases that had been his greatest affliction since he first appeared on earth. Could I, at last, truly see the beginning of the end of my existence on earth?

* Koch, who reported his techniques in 1877, was not the first to employ stains. In 1849, Julius Cohn had used carmine for histological staining and, a year or two later, haematoxylin had been employed for a similar purpose. Carmine had also been used for the first attempts to stain bacteria in about 1869. The first to stain cocci successfully was Carl Weigert (1845-1904) who also used carmine; in 1875 he used methyl violet (an aniline dye, a derivative of coal tar) to stain cocci in animal tissues. – J.G.

ou may wonder, Dr Annandale, why my story stops at this point just over a century ago. The reason is simple: so much has happened in those years that I have been unable to determine which events have increased man's understanding of disease – as, after all, that is my only concern since it is his understanding that will influence my fate. Despite all that has been achieved, man is still groping in the dark in this regard – to which my continued presence here should testify. The achievements (observe that I do not refer to them as progress or advances), particularly in diagnosis and treatment, are a testament to man's ingenuity and industry and have done much to alleviate suffering. But I remain unconvinced that they have brought him any closer to an understanding of the nature of disease. And might what you think you understand perhaps be turned on its head by future generations – as has happened so often in the past?

Some historian, I forget who, once wrote: "Insulted Nature sometimes vindicated her rights".* This, I believe, is the crux of the matter: Nature will always remain a step or two ahead. You have only to look at the history of antibiotics; they have changed the pattern of infective disease and arguably not for the long-term better – the rise of virus diseases could be attributed to their use as more certainly could the development of pathogenicity among previously non-pathogenic organisms. Nature does not like to be disturbed!

If all my years on earth have taught me anything at all, it is that disease is an inescapable part of the human lot. And the past one hundred years, in particular, have persuaded me that Imhotep was wrong in his judgment. The true understanding of disease *does* rest with the gods and is beyond the comprehension of man.

---

* It was Edward Gibbon (1737-1794) of *The Decline and Fall of the Roman Empire* fame. – J.G.

THE
THREE
LETTERS

[James Grenfell had been a classical scholar before reading medicine. He became a professor of clinical pathology. Since retiring, he has devoted himself to his life-long interest – the history of medicine.]

1) From Professor James Grenfell to Dr David Annandale

You have presented me with an awesome task. When you left, you were understandably in a terribly distressed state and didn't make clear why you wanted me to read the manuscript. I cannot believe it was simply for interest's sake – though I was certainly intrigued. I assume, also, you are not looking for an academic critique. So presumably you just want my opinion, but my opinion of what? Of our wandering Babylonian? Of the possibility that his story is true – or a complete fabrication? Of what happened to Hester? Or perhaps my general views on reincarnation and everlasting life on earth?

Before I start, I hope you will forgive me for adding footnotes, some of which are quite elementary, but I cannot overcome my compulsion to make notes on manuscripts – as if I were still teaching my students. To make amends, I have interpreted Baldassare's comments as best I can – his writing is atrocious and he was evidently racing against time to explain the many points he felt called for clarification in the light of subsequent experience.

I think it easiest if I answer my own questions in reverse order. You already know my views on reincarnation and the possibility of an after-life. We used to discuss them at great length during your tutorials. But not even the advancing years have persuaded me that there is life after death, we must all make the best we can of this one – I would never have made a good pre-Renaissance citizen! Nevertheless, I shall probably get an almighty surprise when I wake up one day to find myself parked in purgatory awaiting further instructions. My problem is that, while I think I hold strong beliefs, one of the strongest is that anything is possible; we can rule nothing out.

So where does this get us? Strange as it may seem, I am more inclined to accept the possibility of a permanent residence on earth than that of reincarnation. Don't ask me why. Perhaps it comes from my denial of an after-life. After all, the Wandering Jew and the Flying Dutchman are accepted dramatis personae in western culture, whereas, to me at any rate, reincarnation has more of an eastern flavour. Thus my views on this question get us nowhere.

Now, Hester. That is a different matter entirely. You, if I remember correctly, had worked out the possible explanations for your dream experience without coming to any rational conclusion. Sadly, I have nothing more to suggest. However, when it comes to Hester's behaviour in Alexandria, the only explanation I can offer is one that I trust will not destroy our friendship, although I am sure it must have crossed your mind. I also know it is one you will never accept. It is that Hester had met Baldassare somewhere previously in this life and, seeing him again in Alexandria, let her hormones get the better of her. Having written that, I know with certainty that it could not be so – but it had to be said.

The one sure thing is that, to my mind, you will never see her again. Hester is dead – trust my intuition. Their bodies were probably removed from the wreckage by desert Arabs who then robbed and buried them – or perhaps the authorities removed them for reasons best known to themselves.

Having read Baldassare's manuscript and now writing this letter, I am slowly being driven to the conclusion that his story is true. I admit that any half-competent historian could have regurgitated the facts, but there is something about the way they are told that, for me at any rate, carries the ring of personal experience. As you would expect, given his predicament, he concentrates on man's understanding of disease; I suppose that is why once the start of a discipline has become established he dropped it, although on numerous occasions he must have been witness to subsequent developments.

He has produced a few interpretations that will be novel to modern historians – which I, nevertheless, find completely acceptable. I wish, though, he had enlarged on the spiritual aspects of medicine – touched on in his aside to you during his discussions with Aristotle in which he mentions the Intellect, the Soul and the Heart. That was a metaphysical world, the comprehension of which is lost for ever in our increasingly materialistic world.

As you asked, I have prepared a list of names and dates and, bar one or two – not surprisingly at the beginning – all the characters are historically established. And so far as these are concerned, I can find no inaccuracies in their depiction.

Dear David, I am not being of much help, am I? I think Telesphorus was right when he said that you had been caught up in a slight miscalculation in the timing of events and the best advice I can offer – is no advice at all. I am sorry. It would be easy to say forget the past, marry again and carry on. But that cannot be, can it?

I think I know what you intend to do, and if I am right you will do it whatever I say. That being so, I can only wish you farewell, old friend.

II) From Dr David Annandale to Professor James Grenfell

You are right, of course, except I do not accept that Hester is dead. Quite frankly, I give not a damn for Paul Baldassare. But I care the earth, and more, for Hester and, as you will have guessed, I would give my life for her happiness. (This, incidentally, is not the same as giving my life for hers. This is something people often forget.) I intend to find those two and persuade Baldassare that, in this world, she is rightfully mine, not his – as, indeed she is. Unfortunately for the good of this intention, I am inclined to believe his story, having reread his manuscript many times. He now regards himself as having been unjustly treated from the start and – unless he has pulled the wool over my eyes and is nothing more than a present-day Lothario – I agree with him. So, with that justification, he puts his love for Ishtar above all else. In spite of that, my idea is to convince him that if he returns Hester to her present life, he will restore the status quo ante and will cease to exist.

I am fully aware that I am walking into danger, but I am as nothing without Hester. If I cannot have her, I might as well be dead – and if by chance this should prove the catalyst that brings their strange existences to an end and ensures Hester's happiness in the hereafter (if, as you say, it exists), then so be it.

The reason I now believe Baldassare has suffered an unjust fate – though he seems to have survived nearly five thousand years in remarkably good shape, if my sight of him in Alexandria was anything to go by – is that I agree that mankind will never comprehend the nature of disease. You have only to attend a conference or two to realize that the deeper we probe, the more mysterious does disease become. But maybe this does not matter; perhaps it will be perfectly possible to come to terms with Nature without understanding her innermost workings. I doubt it, though.

Now it is time for me to say my farewell. One way or another, for I now have all the time in the world, I intend to find them. Should I then fail to win Hester back, I pray I may see her for one last fleeting moment before she is united for ever with her Bal-sarra-uzur and hell swallows me up. Farewell, good friend.

III) From Telesphorus to Professor James Grenfell

[This letter did not arrive with the mail in the usual manner. It was delivered separately and the envelope marked: By Hand.]

I will tell the last adventure of your friend David Annandale.

The gods decreed that he should start his search in Alexandria and there I found him, once again, at the crossroads of the ancient world. I went up to him and tugged at his sleeve. It was almost as if this mortal was expecting me.

"Hallo, Telesphorus," he said in a completely matter-of-fact tone.

"Hiere, Dr Annandale," I answered. "I hoped I would meet you here, as I have been sent by my master to take you to him and my mistress."

Tears came into his eyes and he grasped my hand. "Do that," he managed to say.

We travelled the route Alexander had taken. We travelled on foot and we travelled by night, as he had done, but we did so to avoid unwelcome attention from the authorities. We travelled along a chain of hills, rising and falling into valleys until finally a ravine, sparkling from the moonlight playing on the shells underfoot, led us out into a sandy plain hardened by natural salt. And then we came to the oasis at Siwa with its fruit and palm trees, streams and meadow grasses, quails and falcons. We saw it as Alexander saw it that first time.

My master was waiting to greet him. There was no sign of my mistress. The two men shook hands with apparent warmth – I never cease to be amazed at the chivalrous behaviour that can still exist between mortals; I know some gods and ancient heroes who would have been at each other's throats the moment they clapped eyes on their rival.

I cannot tell what passed between them as my master ordered me away. I watched them talking until, quite without warning, a shot rang out from the other side of the clearing and Dr Annandale fell to the ground. My master disappeared into the ruins of the temple while I hurried to Dr Annandale's side. In an instant my mistress, Dr Annandale's Hester, emerged. She dropped to her knees and laid the doctor's head in her lap.

"Oh, my David," she murmured and kissed him on the lips. He opened his eyes, smiled and spoke one sentence. To my amazement it was in Italian.

"Arrestati, sei bello!"

I could not believe what I had heard. The dying man had echoed the words of Goethe's Faust whose soul became forfeit to the devil if he ever became so enamoured of the fleeting moment that he wished it to remain his for ever. (The phrase, when sung in Italian, as in Boito's *Mefistofele* is infinitely more heart-stopping than the original German, "Verweile doch, du bist so schön!" or even the English, "Tarry a while, thou art so fair!" Wouldn't you agree, Professor? But I digress – a failing of mine.)

What happened next, did so on two planes. I shall tell you first what I witnessed. My master appeared and knelt beside Ishtar. They prayed together over the body of Dr Annandale before vanishing once again into the ruins.

As they disappeared, I had my second surprise. The figure of Allatu materialized beside the body.

"I am feared only when men do not know me." She spoke kindly as she took Dr Annandale by the hand and raised him to his feet. "When they know me for what I am and for what I can bring, I am welcomed. Bal-sarra-uzur escaped me and I have made him pay the price through Ishtar's mortality. But both are now gone for ever beyond my reach. And since they owe this to you, a mortal, I bear them no ill-will. Come now, David, I shall carry you across the river to oblivion." And they were gone.

The second version, I can best tell by quoting an item from the same English language newspaper that Dr Annandale had seen in Alexandria. It ran as follows:

"BODIES FOUND IN DESERT. A few weeks ago an army patrol shot and fatally wounded a British national, it was announced yesterday. An official spokesman said the man had entered a restricted area and, when challenged, tried to escape. The body has been returned to England.

"The man was named as Dr David Annandale whose wife, as reported in this newspaper last year, mysteriously disappeared with another doctor after their light aircraft crashed near the Siwa oasis. Dr Annandale is believed to have been making an illegal attempt to solve the mystery when he was killed. He had previously been denied the necessary permission.

"His search had, however, proved successful. His body was lying next to those of Mrs Hester Annandale and the Iraqi doctor, Paul Baldassare. The identification of the two bodies was established only from photographs since they dissolved completely into dust as soon as the attempt was made to move them.

"All that remained were ornate gold chains lying where the woman's wrists, ankles and waist had been. These were sent to the Cairo Museum where an expert stated he had never before seen anything similar.

" 'These are unique,' he said. 'I would guess that they were worn by priestesses at temple ceremonies. They probably date from the third to the fifth dynasties. They will be a valuable addition to the Museum's collection.' "

My master and mistress are at peace now in a world where illusion is no more. And I? Now that my earthly responsibilities are at an end, I shall return to my family on Mount Olympus. So farewell – and I trust, dear Professor, that we, too, may call each other friend.

CHARACTERS AND CHRONOLOGY

[This listing was prepared by James Grenfell at the request of David Annandale. Some of the earlier dates are perforce approximations and of only two of the characters is there no historical record.]

CHAPTER 1 (c.2700 BC - c.1500 BC)
Ebih-Il. Diviner - no historical record
Ishtar. Babylonian goddess - also identified with Astarte
Imhotep. Physician, architect and grand vizier to King Zozer. c.2700 BC. Subsequently deified
Zoser. Pharoah. c.2700 BC
Amenophis I. Pharoah. c.1500 BC
Seneb. Scribe - no historical record
Astarte. Goddess of Eastern Mediterranean regions - also identified with Ishtar

CHAPTER 2 (c.1500 BC)
Tammuz. Babylonian/Syrian god - also identified with Adonis
Allatu. Goddess of the land of the dead in Eastern Mediterranean regions
Hammurapi, King of Babylon. 1792 BC - 1750 BC

CHAPTER 3 (c.1200 BC - c.425 BC)
Asklepios. Greek god of medicine
Telesphorus. Mythological son of Asklepios

Panacea and Hygeia. Goddess daughters of Asklepios
Pindar. Greek poet. *c.*552 BC - *c.*442 BC
[Thucydides. Historian. *c.*470 BC - 399 BC]
Hippocrates. Physician. 460 BC - 370 BC
Pythagoras. Scientist. *c.*582 BC - *c.*507 BC

CHAPTER 4 (370 BC – 321 BC)
Aristotle. Philosopher scientist. 384 BC - 322 BC
Alexander the Great, King of Macedonia. 356 BC - 323 BC
Philip II, King of Macedonia. Father of Alexander. 382 BC - 336 BC
Plato. Philosopher. 427 BC - 347 BC
Hermeias, King of Mysia. *fl.*360 BC
Ptolemy. Ruler and then king of Egypt. *c.*367 BC - 283 BC
Hephaestion. Friend of Alexander. d.324 BC
Olympias. Mother of Alexander. d. *c.*321 BC
Dinocrates. Architect to Alexander the Great. *fl.*332 BC
Darius III, King of Persia. d.330 BC
Oxyartes. Ruler of Bactria. *fl.*325 BC
Roxana. Daughter of Oxyartes and wife of Alexander. d. *c.*321 BC

CHAPTER 5 (321 BC - 30 BC)
Herophilus. Anatomist. 335 BC - 280 BC
Erasistratus. Physiologist. 310 BC - 250 BC
Chrysippus of Cnidos. Greek physician. *fl.*340 BC
Cicero. Roman writer and statesman. 106 BC - 43 BC
Themison. Philosopher of the Methodist school. *fl.*50 BC
Democritus. Philosopher. *c.*460 BC - 362 BC
Empedocles. Greek scientist, philosopher and poet. *c.* 460 BC

CHAPTER 6 (166 - 169)
Gaius Julius Caesar. Sole ruler of Rome - marking the end of the
    Republic. *c.*101 BC - 44 BC
Claudius Galen. Physician. 129 - *c.*200-216
Aurelius Cornelius Celsus. Aristocratic lay compiler of, and
    commentator upon, available medical literature. 25 BC - 50 AD
Ovid. Poet. 43 BC - 17 BC
Virgil. Epic poet. 70 BC - 19 BC
Marcus Aurelius. Last of the Five Good Emperors of Rome. 121 - 180

Lucius Verus. Co-emperor with Marcus Aurelius. 130 - 175
Statius Priscus. Roman general. *fl.*165
Avidius Cassius. Roman general. *c.*131 - 169
Panthea. Syrian mistress of Lucius. *fl.*165
Apollonius of Chalcedon. Stoic philosopher. *fl.*140
Aurelius Commodus. Son of Marcus Aurelius; co-emperor and
    successor. 161 - 192 (assassinated)
Annius Verus. Son of Marcus Aurelius. 162 - 169
Annia Galeria Faustina. Wife of Marcus Aurelius. *c.*130 - 175

CHAPTER 7 (169 - 177)
Annia Aurelia Galeria Lucilla. Daughter of Marcus Aurelius and
    wife of Lucius. 150 - *c.*182
Tiberius Claudius Pompeianus. Second husband of Lucilla. *fl.*169
Lucian of Samosata in Syria. Roman satirist. *c.*125 - *c.*190
Praxagoras of Cos. Philosopher scientist. *fl.*335 BC
Pitholaus. Tutor to Commodus. *fl.*174
Martius Verus. Roman general. *fl.*175

CHAPTER 8 (c.400 - c.900)
Magnus of Emesa in Syria and/or Nisibis in Mesopotamia. Compiler
    of works of Galen. *fl.* 370

CHAPTER 9 (c.900 - 1037)
Mohamed. The Prophet. *c.*570 - 632
al-Ma'mun. 7th Abbasid caliph. d.833
Qusta ibn Luqa. Christian polymath and translator. d.912
Hunayn ibn Ishaq. Nestorian priest and translator. 808 - 873
Rhazes (Abu Bakr Mohamed ibn Zakariyya al-Razi). Physician.
    *c.*865 - 925
Pedanius (Pedacius) Dioscorides. Turkish physician in the Roman
    army of Nero. Avid collector and recorder of medicines, mainly
    herbal. *fl.*60
Avicenna (Abu Ali al-Hasayn ibn-Sina). Physician. 980 - 1037

CHAPTER 10 (c.1037 - c.1330)
Constantinus Africanus. Monk, scholar, translator. *c.*1020 - 1097

Mondino de Luzzi (Mundinus). Anatomist and surgeon at Bologna. 1270 - 1326

Alessandra Gilliani. Anatomical prosector and assistant to Mondino. *fl.*1300

Aretaeus of Cappadocia. Physician. *fl.*2nd - 3rd century AD

CHAPTER 11 (c.1330 - 1348)

Fiammetta. Boccaccio's affectionate name for Maria d'Aquino, natural daughter of Robert the Wise, King of Naples. d.1348

Giovanni Boccaccio. Author of, inter alia, the *Decameron*. 1313 - 1375

St Francis of Assisi. Called Francis by his father, Pietro di Bernardone, but baptized John. Canonized two years after his death. 1182 - 1226

Giotto di Bendone. Artist. c.1267 - 1337

Cimabue, the nickname of Cenni di Pepo. Artist. c.1240 - c.1302

Simone Martini. Siennese artist. c.1284 - 1344

Lorenzetti brothers. Siennese artists. Pietro, c.1280 - c.1348. Ambrogio, *fl.*1320. It is possible that both died during the Black Death

Aesculapius. Roman god of medicine. Identified with the Greek Asklepios

CHAPTER 12 (1348 - 1516)

Geber (Jabir ibn-Hayyan). Arabian chemist and alchemist. *fl.*776

Juan Ponce de Léon. Spanish explorer and discoverer of Florida in 1513. c.1460 - 1521

Johannes Tritheim (Trithemius). Ecclesiastic and alchemist. 1462 - 1516

Moses Maimonides. Physician-philosopher of the Western Caliphate. 1135 - 1204

CHAPTER 13 (Second quarter 16th century)

Paracelsus (Theophrastus Philippus Aureolus Bombastus von Hohenheim), Swiss alchemist and physician (though whether qualified is uncertain). Bombastus was his father's family name, but he adopted the name of Paracelsus (superior to Celsus) in about 1529. 1493 - 1541

Joannes Oporinus. Swiss printer; Professor of Greek at Basle University; one-time amanuensis to Paracelsus. 1507 - 1568

Andreas Vesalius (André Wesel). Belgian anatomist; Professor of Anatomy at Padua. 1514 - 1564

Jan Stephan van Calcar (Kalcar). Artist; student of Titian. 1499 - 1546

Leonardo da Vinci. One of the greatest figures of the Italian Renaissance. 1452 - 1519

Desiderius Erasmus. Dutch scholar and humanist. c.1466 - 1536

The identity of the Benedictine monk is obscure. He may have been Johann Estchenreuter who wrote under the pseudonym of Basil Valentine. fl.1500

Archbishop Ernst of Salzburg. fl.1540

[Averroës (abu-al-Walid Muhammad ibn-Ahmad ibn-Rushd). Arabian philosopher and physician of the Western Caliphate. 1126-1198]

Sylvius (Jacques Dubois). Parisian anatomist. 1478 - 1555

Masaccio (Tommaso di Giovanni di Simone Guidi). Florentine artist. 1401 - 1428

Filippo Brunelleschi. Italian architect. 1377 - 1446

Johann Gutenberg (Gensfleisch). German printer; inventor of moveable metal type. c.1400 - 1468

Charles V, Holy Roman Emperor. 1500 - 1558

Philip II, King of Spain. 1527 - 1598

CHAPTER 14 (Second half 16th century – first half 17th century)

William Harvey. English physician; discovered the circulation of the blood. 1578 - 1657

Robert Boyle. Seventh son of the Earl of Cork. Chemist; intensely interested in medicine, especially experimental; obtained a medical degree in 1665. A founder of the Royal Society. 1627 - 1691

Giambattista Canano. Professor of Anatomy at Ferrara. 1515 - 1579

Amatus Lusitanus (Juan Rodriguez). Anatomist. 1511 - 1568

Heironymus Fabricius ab Aquapendente. Professor of Anatomy at Padua. 1533 - 1619

Andrea Cesalpino. Italian physician. 1519 - 1603

Pope Clement VIII. 1536 - 1605

Salomon Alberti. Professor of Medicine at Wittenberg. *fl.*1585

Matteo Realdo Colombo. Vesalius's prosector at Padua; later, Professor of Anatomy at Rome. 1516 - 1559

Jean Riolan the Younger. Professor of Anatomy at Paris. 1577 - 1657

René Descartes. French mathematician and philosopher. 1596 - 1650

Christina, Queen of Sweden from 1632 to 1654 when she abdicated. 1626 - 1689

CHAPTER 15 (Second half 17th century)

Marcello Malpighi. Italian physician and microscopist; Professor of Medicine at Bologna, Pisa and Messina. 1628 - 1694

Socrates. Athenian philosopher. *c.*469 - 399 BC

Giovanni Alfonso Borelli. Italian mathematician. 1608 - 1679

Antonj van Leeuwenhoek. Dutch cloth merchant turned microscopist. 1632 - 1723

Thomas Sydenham. English physician (the "English Hippocrates"). 1624 - 1689

CHAPTER 16 (18th century)

Théophile Bonet. Swiss physician. 1620 - 1689

Duc de Longueville. *fl.*1670

Giovanni Battista Morgagni. Professor of Anatomy at Padua. 1682 - 1771

Antonio Maria Valsalva. Professor of Anatomy at Padua. 1666 - 1723

Marie-François-Xavier Bichat. French anatomist. 1771 - 1802

Jean-Nicolas Corvisart des Marets. French physician. 1755 - 1821

CHAPTER 17 (1802-1815)

Napoleon Bonaparte. 1769-1821

Dominique Jean Larrey. French military surgeon. 1766 - 1842

Luigi Cherubini. Italian composer. 1760 - 1842

Euripides. Greek tragic poet. 481 BC - 406 BC

Julie-Angélique Scio (née Le Grand). French operatic soprano. 1768 - 1807

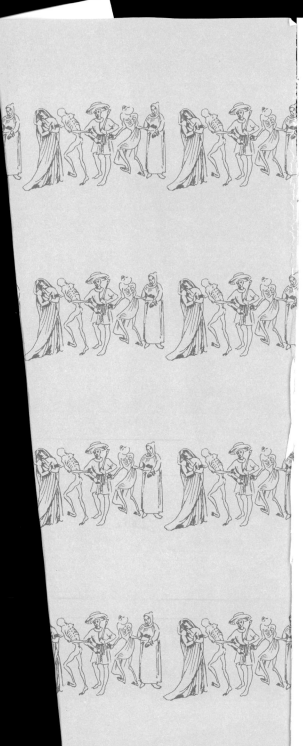

Charlotte Elisabeth Larrey (née Laville). Wife of Dominique Jean. 1770 - 1842

Etienne Scio. French violinist; husband of Julie-Angélique. 1766 - 1796

Michel Ney, Duke of Elchingen, Prince of the Moskova. 1769 - 1815

Pierre François Percy. Surgeon-in-Chief of the Grande Armée at its inception. 1754 - 1825

Wolfgang Amadeus Mozart. Austrian composer. 1756 - 1791

Christophe Willibald von Gluck. German composer. 1714 - 1787

Frederick William III, King of Prussia. 1770 - 1840

Alexander I of Russia. 1777 - 1825

[Alexander Pope. English poet. 1688 - 1744]

CHAPTER 18 (1815 - 1826)

Leopold Auenbrugger. Austrian physician. 1722 - 1809

René-Théophile-Hyacinth Laennec. French physician. 1781 - 1826

Sir John Forbes. Scottish physician; practised in England; Physician to the Court of Queen Victoria. 1787 - 1861

[John Keats. English poet. 1795 - 1821]

CHAPTER 19 (Mid-19th century - 1881)

Francesco Redi. Italian naturalist. 1626 - 1697

Louis Pasteur. French chemist; Director of the Institut Pasteur. 1822 - 1895

Theodor Schwann. Professor of Anatomy and Physiology at Liège. 1810 - 1882

Jakob Friedrich Gustav Henle. Professor of Anatomy at Zurich, Heidelberg and Göttingen. 1809 - 1885

Robert Koch. German physician. Professor of Hygeine and Bacteriology at the University of Berlin. 1843 - 1910

Ferdinand Julius Cohn. Professor of Botany at Breslau; bacteriologist. 1828 - 1898

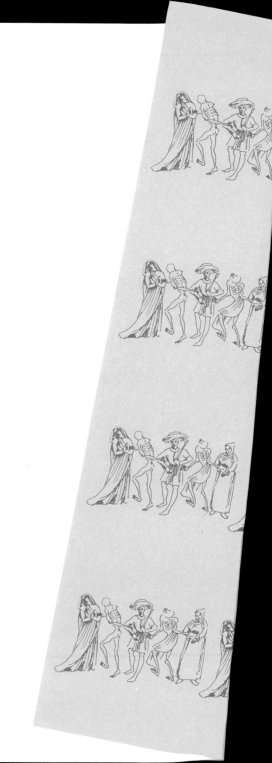